D1560533

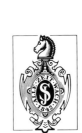

Bruce Pomeranz Gabriel Stux (Eds.)

Scientific Bases of
Acupuncture

With Contributions by
Jisheng Han B. Pomeranz Kang Tsou C. Takeshige
J. M. Chung D. Le Bars J.-C. Willer T. de Broucker
L. Villanueva R. S. S. Cheng M. H. M. Lee M. Ernst
and G. A. Ulett

With 79 Figures

Springer-Verlag
Berlin Heidelberg New York London Paris Tokyo

Prof. Bruce Pomeranz M. D., Ph. D.
Dept. of Physiology (Faculty of Medicine)
Dept. of Zoology (Faculty of Arts and Science)
University of Toronto
25, Harbord St., Toronto M5S1A1
Ontario, Canada

Dr. med. Gabriel Stux M. D.
Acupuncture Centrum
Goltsteinstrasse 26, D-4000 Düsseldorf
Federal Republic of Germany

ISBN 3-540-19335-9 Springer-Verlag Berlin Heidelberg New York
ISBN 0-387-19335-9 Springer-Verlag New York Berlin Heidelberg

Typesetting, printing and binding: Appl, Wemding
2119/3140/543210 - Printed on acid-free paper

Preface

Serious basic research on acupuncture began in 1976 when the acupuncture endorphin hypothesis was postulated. In the ensuing twelve years (1976–1988), a critical mass of rigorous research on acupuncture has accumulated, necessitating this book to bring it all together. Moreover, the growth of acupuncture world-wide, to the point where there are over one million practitioners doing acupuncture, makes it important to disseminate this important research data. Finally, a comprehensive book was needed for legislators, hospital administrators, insurance companies and government agencies, etc., to help them make decisions on a more rational basis; many regulations made in 1976 should be revised in 1988 based on 12 years of new data!

As a result of this need to prepare a book, the editors arranged a conference in Düsseldorf, Germany, to coincide with the 1987 IASP (International Association for the Study of Pain) Congress to which leading researchers from around the world were invited to present review papers on acupuncture and to discuss the state of the field. As an outgrowth of this successful conference, each of the participants was asked to write a review chapter for this anthology. In this chapter, they were asked to summarize the research from their laboratory and to correlate it with the broader literature on acupuncture.

As can be seen from this comprehensive, multi-authored book, there is an enormous amount of rigorous research into the mechanisms of acupuncture. Indeed, we know more about acupuncture analgesia mechanisms than many conventional medical procedures. Perhaps the time has come to stop calling acupuncture an "experimental procedure".

Summer 1988   The Editors

Table of Contents

List of Contributors

Dr. Richard S. S. Cheng M. D., Ph. D., Director Pain Clinic St. Josephs Hospital and Bathurst Pain Clinic, 800 Bathurst Street, Toronto, Canada

Prof. Jin Mo Chung Ph. D., Marine Biomedical Institute and Departments of Anatomy & Neurosciences and of Physiology & Biophysics, University of Texas Medical Branch, 200 University Boulevard, Galveston, Texas 77550, USA

Dr. Thomas de Broucker Ph. D., Dept. Physiol., Lab. Neurophysiol., Faculté Médecine Pitié-Salpêtrière, 91, Bd. de l'Hôpital, 75013 Paris, France

Monique Ernst M. D., Ph. D., Chronic Pain Unit, New York University Medical Center, Goldwater Memorial Hospital, Franklin D. Roosevelt Island, and Department of Psychiatry, Beth Israel Medical Center, New York, N. Y. 10044, USA

Prof. Jisheng Han M. D., Neuroscience Research Center and Chairman Department of Physiology, Beijing Medical University, Beijing 100083, China

Prof. Daniel Le Bars, INSERM U-161, 2, rue d'Alesia, 75014 Paris, France

Prof. Mathew H. M. Lee M. D., MPH, FACP, Director of Clinical Rehabilitation Medicine, New York University, Goldwater Memorial Hospital, Franklin D. Roosevelt Island, New York, N. Y. 10044, USA

Prof. Bruce Pomeranz M. D., Ph. D., Departments of Zoology and Physiology, University of Toronto, 25 Harbord Street, Toronto M551A, Canada

Dr. Gabriel Stux M. D., Acupuncture Center Düsseldorf, Goltsteinstr. 26, 4000 Düsseldorf, Federal Republic of Germany

Prof. Chifuyu Takeshige M. D., Department of Physiology, Dean of School of Medicine, Showa University, 1-5-8 Hatanodai, Shinagawa, Tokyo, Japan 142

Prof. Kang Tsou M. D., Department of Pharmacology, Shanghai Institute of Materia Medica, Chinese Academy of Sciences, 319 Yue-Yang Road, Shanghai 200031, China

Prof. George A. Ulett M. D., Clinical Professor of Psychiatry, St. Louis University School of Medicine. Director Department of Psychiatry, Deaconess Hospital, 6150 Oakland Avenue, St. Louis, MO 63139, USA

Dr. Luis Villanueva Ph. D., INSERM U-161, 2, rue d'Alesia, 75014 Paris, France

Prof. Jean-Claude Willer M. D., DSc., Dept. Physiol., Lab. Neurophysiol., Faculté Médecine Pitié-Salpêtrière, 91, Bd. de l'Hôpital, 75013 Paris, France

Introduction

Gabriel Stux and Bruce Pomeranz

Acupuncture is experiencing a renaissance both in China and world wide with over 1 million practitioners using it. In the 19th century, acupuncture declined in China after 2500 years of widespread use. This is attributed to western influences and the degeneration of Chinese culture as a result of foreign Manchu rule. After 1949, when the People's republic was founded, Mao Zedong encouraged the practice of acupuncture which marks the beginning of the current renaissance. Academies of Chinese medicine were established in Beijing, Shanghai, Nanking and other major cities. Western style medical schools such as Beijing University and Shanghai First Medical School also began to research into the basic mechanisms of acupuncture. Unfortunately, their failure to publish in English, and the general distrust of Chinese science by western scientists and physicians, kept this new information from disseminating. However, one phenomenon caught the eye of westerners: the development of acupuncture anesthesia for surgical operations. Spectacular documentory films showing awake patients having surgery under the influence of acupuncture, awakened the interest of the western medical world. As a result acupuncture for the treatment of chronic pain was gradually introduced into many western pain clinics starting in 1972, after Nixon opened up ties with China. In the USSR acupuncture was introduced in the 1950's because of close political ties with China. Europe had several schools of acupuncture since the 1930's, but the major impetus for acupuncture's spread in the west came after Nixon's visit to China.

However skepticism remained high. How could a needle in the hand possibly relieve a toothache? Because such phenomena did not fit into the existing knowledge of physiology, scientists and clinicians were skeptical. Many explained it by the well-known placebo effect [11]. In 1955 Beecher had shown that, while morphine relieved pain in majority of patients, sugar injections (placebo) reduced pain in 30% of patients who believed they were receiving morphine [2]. Thus many pain physiologists in the 1970's assumed that AA worked by the placebo (psychological) effect. However, there were several problems with this idea. How does one explain its widespread use in veterinary medicine and in pediatrics? Moreover studies in which patients were given psychological tests for suggestibility did not show a good correlation between acupuncture analgesia (AA) and suggestibility (see review of Ulett in this volume, and [5]). Hypnosis has also been ruled out as an explanation as studies show that hypnotic analgesia and AA respond differently to naloxone, AA being blocked and hypnosis being unaffected by this endorphin antagonist [1, 3].

1

In addition to the lack of a plausible mechanism to explain AA, skeptics were concerned about the anecdotal nature of acupuncture claims. Despite the huge size of the anecdotal database (one quarter of the world's population had been using acupuncture for 2500 years) skeptics were calling for controlled clinical studies to prove the efficacy of acupuncture.

A growing body of research published in the past 12 years shows that AA is very effective in treating chronic pain, helping from 55% to 85% of patients [4, 8, 10], which compares favourably with potent drugs. Moreover the evidence shows that in placebo control groups only 30% of cases were helped proving that AA is more effective than placebo and that AA is a real physical effect (see appendix for details). In addition to the clinical studies which prove efficacy, the only way to overcome the deep skepticism towards acupuncture was to establish credible physiological mechanisms of action.

The breakthrough came in 1976, soon after the discovery of endorphins. Two groups, one studying human volunteers [6], the other working on animals [7] showed that naloxone (an endorphin antagonist) blocked AA. The acupuncture-endorphin hypothesis which emerged proposed that AA is a result of peripheral nerve stimulation which sends impulses to the brain to release endorphins and causes analgesia [9]. This hypothesis, more than any other, has stimulated research in dozens of laboratories on 4 continents. A recent review summarizes over 200 papers in the western literature on this subject [9].

Because of the extensive literature which has now accumulated, it was decided to ask leading scientists to each write a chapter reviewing their own research and related papers.

Prof. Jisheng Han, Chairman of the Physiology Department, Beijing Medical University (China), considered to be one of China's leading neuroscientists, and is world renowned for his animal studies on acupuncture mechanisms. In his work he showed that electrical stimulation of needles released different endorphin compounds at different pulse frequencies. Thus with EA at 4 Hz enkephalins were activated while at 100 Hz dynorphins were released. Very elegant experiments were used to prove these facts. For examples antibodies to enkephalins injected intrathecally onto the spinal cord of rats blocked acupuncture analgesia produced by 4 Hz EA, while antibodies to dynorphins blocked 100 Hz EA.

Prof. Kang Tsou, Chairman Department of Pharmacology at Shanghai Institute of Materia Medica, Chinese Academy of Science, is China's most renowned endorphin researcher. Using advanced molecular biology techniques (eg DNA hybridization) he showed that the messanger RNA involved in making endorphins was elevated in the rat brain 1 hour after EA, an effect which lasted 48 hours. This suggests that long term analgesia from acupuncture could be caused by increased synthesis of endorphins.

Prof. Bruce Pomeranz, Professor of Physiology and Zoology at University of Toronto (Canada) has published 42 papers on neural effects of acupuncture in animals and humans; his laboratory was one of the first to show that acupuncture analgesia was mediated by endorphins. He began his work with spinal cord experiments in anesthetized animals. Recording from single cells involved in nociceptive transmission from spinal cord to brain he showed that EA blocked the message and that this effect was prevented by naloxone, the endorphin antagonist. In

2

another series of experiments he showed that intrathecal naltrexone only blocked when injected before acupuncture treatment began, but could not block analgesia if given after completion of the acupuncture treatment. He has recent publications suggesting that acupuncture is not merely useful for analgesia and reported that EA speeds up nerve regeneration in the leg of adult rats after nerve injury. Acupuncture is in widespread use in China for treatment of neurological diseases which have no pain components. Finally in his review he described a transcutaneous electrical nerve stimulation (TENS) device which he developed to give patients "De Qi" sensations from deep muscle nerves. This device produces much more effective analgesia in chronic pain patients than either conventional TENS or standard EA, which he showed by controlled studies.

Dr. Richard Cheng, Director of the Pain Clinic at St. Josephs Hospital in Toronto (Canada) showed the importance of frequency of stimulation (compare Prof. Han above). His results indicate that in mice, 4 Hz pulses work through endorphin mechanisms, while 200 Hz stimulation is mediated by monoamines (serotonin and norepinephrine).

Prof. Jin Mo Chung, Professor of Physiology at University of Texas in Galveston (USA) and a senior scientist in the renowned pain laboratory of Prof. W. D. Willis at the Marine Biomedical Institute, performed a series of elegant experiments on decerebrate spinalized animals, showing that small diameter myelinated peripheral nerves (A delta and type III) produced analgesia against heat pain, while causing no effect on pinch pain or "touch". Presumably this suggests that pain from unmyelinated "C" fibres is more easily suppressed than pain from "A delta" fibres by acupuncture-like stimulation.

Prof. Chifuyu Takeshige, Dean of Medicine at Showa University in Tokyo (Japan), described an "Analgesia Inhibitory System" influenced by specific acupuncture points. In a series of 10 elegant papers (published in Japanese) Prof. Takeshige's group reported on an "Analgesia Inhibitory System" which is activated by giving acupuncture to points in the ventral abdominal region of the rat. Lesions placed anywhere along the brain circuitry of this inhibitory system unmasked the ventral abdominal points, enabling these sites to produce acupuncture analgesia which they cannot do in intact rats. All together Prof. Takeshige's group has published over 50 papers on acupuncture mechanisms (in Japanese). He also reviewed some recent experiments showing that acupuncture can overcome muscle fatigue in rats undergoing repetitive muscle activation. This is an additional example of non-analgesic properties of acupuncture.

Another review was written by Prof. D. Le Bars, Prof. J. C. Willer, Dr. T. de Broucker and L. Villanueva of University of Paris (France) (from the renowned pain group of J. M. Besson at INSERM). It was titled "Neurophysiological Mechanisms Involved in Pain Relieving Effect of Counterirritation and Related Techniques Including Acupuncture". This review was in two parts. The first summarized the results from Prof. Le Bars' group in rats, showing that pain in one part of the body inhibits pain responses in another part; when observed on spinal cord dorsal horn wide dynamic range neurons this effect has been called DNIC (diffuse non specific inhibitory control); when observed in behaving rats, or with flexor withdrawal reflexes in humans it is called "counterirritation". Whether or not DNIC is a model for acupuncture is unclear, as unmyelinated "C" fibres are activated for the conditioning stimulus, whereas acupuncture generally activates small myelinated "A delta" and type III muscle afferents. The famous "De Qi" sensation produced by acupuncture is a mild ache and not frank pain. Also the time course of DNIC is a matter of controversy; it shows a rapid onset and short after-effect, starting immediately and lasting only several minutes after conditioning stimulus ends. Acupuncture has a much longer induction time and after-effect, taking 5 to 30 minutes to get going, and outlasting the treatment by 20 min to several hours.

In the second part of the review the counterirritation experiments conducted in humans had a much more appropriate time course for a model of acupuncture than the DNIC experiments in rats. Moreover, the human experiments were very convincing because of the beautiful correlation of flexor reflex suppression (measured by sural evoked reflex EMGs from biceps femoris) and psychophysical measures of sensory analgesia produced by counterirritation. The subjects dipped their arm into hot water (above 45 °C) several minutes to produce counterirritation. This produced analgesia which had after-effects lasting 10–15 minutes. The effect was blocked by naloxone (pretreatment), and was absent in paraplegic patients.

Prof. Mathew Lee, Professor of Rehabilitation Medicine at New York University (USA), wrote a review on "Clinical and Research Observations on Acupuncture Analgesia and Thermography". In the first part of the review it was shown that strong (above pain threshold) EA of LI.4 (1st dorsal interosseus muscle of the hand) produced a 30% increased in the discomfort threshold for tooth electrical stimulation in normal volunteers, an effect which took 40 min to reach its peak. Naloxone was able to partially block this effect when given 10 min after onset of the EA treatment.

Perhaps, it was the second half of his review which was most novel as it dealt with a non-analgesic property of acupuncture: the effect of acupuncture on the autonomic control of skin circulation. The elegant design involved measurement of skin temperature of hands, feet and face using infrared colour thermography. Acupuncture treatments were given to normal volunteers in either LI.4 (1st dorsal interosseus muscle) or St.36 (tibialis anterior muscle) by one of two methods: either manual twirling of the needles manual acupuncture MA to produce mild painful sensations, or EA at 1 Hz at below pain threshold. Whereas MA caused marked vasodilatation in all regions from either acupuncture site, the results from EA were less consistent. Could this difference be attributed to intensity of stimulation? It seems that consistent results were only obtained when "De Qi" was obtained (compare Prof. Pomeranz's TENS study on humans). Prof. Lee thus showed convincing evidence that acupuncture is not just useful for analgesia, but should be studied further for its effects on autonomic function.

Prof. George Ulett, Professor of Psychiatry at St. Louis University School of Medicine and Director of Psychiatry Deaconess Hospital (USA), wrote a review entitled "Studies Supporting the Concept of Physiological Acupuncture". His work covered a broad range of topics. He showed that EA raised white blood cell counts in normal human subjects by 40%; however there was no significant difference between needling acupuncture points and non-acupuncture sites. The stimulus intensity was kept below pain threshold, and hence it would be interesting to

4

repeat the experiments while producing "De Qi". Clearly more research on non-analgesic effects of acupuncture is needed. In another important study Prof. Ulett showed that acupuncture is as effective as morphine or hypnosis in suppressing experimental pain in human volunteers. Since hypnotic susceptibility did not correlate with acupuncture success rate, the two are not the same phenomenon (a result confirmed by others using naloxone antagonists which block acupuncture but not hypnotic analgesia).

Unfortunately several additional researchers who were invited to attend the Düsseldorf Acupuncture Symposium (1987) could not come because of conflicts in their schedule. Professors David Mayer, Lars Terenius, Sven Andersson, Bengt Sjölund, Peter Hand, and Manfred Zimmermann were thus unable to contribute to this volume. We hope to include their contributions in later anthologies.

References

1. Barber J, Mayer DJ (1977) Evaluation of the efficacy and neural mechanism of a hypnotic analgesia procedure in experimental and clinical dental pain. Pain 4: 41–48
2. Beecher HK (1955) Placebo analgesia in human volunteers. J Am Med Assoc 159: 1602–1606
3. Goldstein A, Hilgard EF (1975) Failure of the opiate antagonist naloxone to modify hypnotic analgesia. Proc Natl Acad Sci USA 72: 2041–2043
4. Lewith GT, Field J, Machin D (1983) Acupuncture compared with placebo in post-herpetic pain. Pain 17: 361–368
5. Liao SJ (1978) Recent advances in the understanding of acupuncture. Yale J Biol Med 51: 55–65
6. Mayer DJ, Price DD, Raffi A (1977) Antagonism of acupuncture analgesia in man by the narcotic antagonist naloxone. Brain Res 121: 368–372
7. Pomeranz B, Chiu D (1976) Naloxone blocks acupuncture analgesia and causes hyperalgesia: endorphin is implicated. Life Sci 19: 1757–1762
8. Richardson PH, Vincent CA (1986) Acupuncture for the treatment of pain: a review of evaluative research. Pain 24: 15–40
9. Stux G, Pomeranz B (1987) Acupuncture – textbook and atlas. Springer Verlag, Heidelberg
10. Vincent CA, Richardson PH (1986) The evaluation of therapeutic acupuncture: concepts and methods. Pain 24: 1–13
11. Wall PD (1972) An eye on the needle. New Sci July 20, pp 129–131

Central Neurotransmitters and Acupuncture Analgesia

Jisheng Han

Neuroscience Research Center and Department of Physiology, Beijing Medical University, Beijing 100083, China

In a review article entitled "Neurochemical Basis of Acupuncture Analgesia" [1] I summarized the relevant information up to 1980 on a worldwide basis. The present review will cover only studies performed in the 1980s in my laboratory which are relevant to central neurotransmitters mediating acupuncture analgesia (AA). To make the review brief there are no lengthy discussions on each topic. The reader is referred to original articles for relevant comments.

Animal Models for Acupuncture Analgesia

The study was started in 1965 by observing the basic phenomena of AA in healthy human volunteers and in patients with or without neurological disorders [2]. To study the mechanisms of AA, rabbits [3-5], rats [6-8], and occasionally mice [9] were used as animal models. For nociceptive tests, I recorded the latency of the tail flick response [7-9] or head jerk response [3-5] induced by radiant heat applied to the skin of the tail or nostril region, or the threshold of vocalization in response to subcutaneous electrical stimulation [6].

There has been some controversy over the category of afferent fibers carrys signals from acupuncture or electroacupuncture (EA) stimulation, especially over the involvement of C fibers in the afferent nerves. To abolish C-fiber input capsaicin was applied topically on the sciatic nerves of the rat. Blockade of C-fiber transmission was verified by the disappearance of the C component in the composite nerve impulse recordings and by the abolishment of the withdrawal of the hind limb in response to noxious heating applied to the hind leg region. EA stimulation was then adminstered through stainless steel needles inserted into the St. 36 Zusanli point (located below the knee joint) and Sp. 6 Sanyinjiao point (in front of the Achilles tendon). No significant difference in the effect of EA analgesia was found between the capsaicin group and the control group in which the vehicle (tween 80) was applied on both sciatic nerves. The results imply that C fibers are not indispensible for the transmission of signals aroused by EA stimulation [10].

Concerning the question of whether the neuronal circuit of AA resides in the spinal cord, the effect of AA in rats with spinal transection made at T3 level was tested. The analgesic effect induced by EA (frequency from 2 Hz up to 100 Hz, intensity from 3 V up to 9 V) applied to the hind legs, as assessed by the tail flick latency (TFL), was almost totally abolished in the spinal animal, although the lumbosacral cord remained intact for the intraspinal connection between the neural

7

structures receiving acupuncture input from the hind legs and that controlling the tail flick response. The results suggest that a suprasegmental connection is cardinal for the mediation of AA in this rat model [11].

One of the basic phenomena common in humans and in laboratory animals is that while most of the individuals respond to acupuncture stimulation with an increase in pain threshold (responders), a certain percentage fail to do so (nonresponders). The incidence of nonresponders, usually in the range of 15%–20% in rats, tends to increase in the spring season (data to be published). The underlying mechanisms are as yet unknown. What is clear is that a good correlation exists between the analgesic response to EA and that to morphine (3 mg/kg, s.c.; $r = 0.76$, $n = 113$, $P < 0.001$) [12]. In other words, a good responder to EA is also a good responder to morphine, and vice versa. Since it has been suggested that both EA and morphine release endogenous opioids, a decreased ability to release opioids and an increased capability of releasing endogenous antagonists to opioids might be the mechanisms underlying the nonresponsiveness to EA and morphine (see below).

Classical Neurotransmitters Involved in Acupuncture Analgesia

5-Hydroxytryptamine

A series of studies were published in the 1970s to document the importance of central 5-hydroxytryptamine (5-HT) in mediating AA in rabbits [13, 14], rats [15, 16], mice [16a], and humans [17]. In recent years attempts have been made to identify its site of action in the CNS and to characterize the necessary parameters of EA to activate the 5-HT system.

To clarify the relative importance of 5-HT in the brain and in the spinal cord, 5-hydroxytryptophan (5-HTP), the precursor of 5-HT, and cinanserin, the 5-HT receptor blocker, were injected either intracerebroventricularly (ICV) or intrathecally (ITh) into the rat. Cinanserin produced a 66% and 53% decrease in the effect of AA after ICV and ITh injection, respectively, whereas 5-HTP produced a 54% and 47% increase. The results indicate that 5-HT released in either the brain or the spinal cord seems to play an equally important part in mediating AA [18].

Further studies were performed to identify the site of action in various brain nuclei. The effect of AA was significantly attenuated when cinanserin was microinjected bilaterally into the nucleus accumbens [19], habenula [19], amygdala [20], and periaqueductal gray matter (PAG) [21]. Administration of the same dose of cinanserin (2 µg) to the vicinity of the four nuclei produced no significant effects, showing site specificity of the 5-HT action.

It is interesting to note that while focal injection of cinanserin was very effective in blocking analgesia produced by EA or by a small dose of morphine (2 and 4 mg/kg, SC), it failed to do so when the dose of morphine was increased to 6 mg/kg or more [21]. The former, therefore, seems to be mediated by serotonergic pathways, whereas the latter must be the direct effect of morphine on morphine receptors in nociceptive neurons.

Administration of cinanserin to any of the four brain nuclei mentioned above produced to significant changes in the pain threshold of the rabbit [18-21]. However, ITh injection of cinanserin in the rat produced a significant decrease in pain threshold [22], suggesting a tonic release of 5-HT in the spinal cord of the rat.

In view of the notion that analgesia produced by EA of different parameters (low versus high frequency and/or intensity, etc.) might be mediated by different neurochemical mechanisms (see below), I decided to study the role of 5-HT in analgesia produced by EA of different frequencies (2, 15, 100 Hz continuous, or 2-15 Hz alternate) and different intensities (3 and 9 V). Intraperitoneal (IP) injection of the 5-HT synthesis blocker parachlorophenylalanine (PCPA) methylester, 320 mg/kg, produced an almost equal degree (84%-90%) of suppression of EA analgesia, no matter which frequency and intensity were used [23]. This is in contrast to the situation in the opioid system, in which different opioid peptides are released in response to EA of different frequencies (see below).

Catecholamines

From the studies performed in the 1970s an apparently clear cut, yet oversimplified impression arose that catecholamines (CAs) and 5-HT play opposite roles in mediating AA: AA is facilitated by 5-HT [13-17] and suppressed by central norepinephrine (NE) [24, 25]. However, detailed studies revealed that NE seems to play contradictory roles in the brain and spinal cord. Thus, dihydroxyphenylserine (DOPS), a direct precursor of NE, suppressed AA in the brain (-65%) and potentiated AA in the spinal cord ($+37\%$); the alpha-adrenoceptor blocker phentolamine, in contrast, potentiated AA in the brain ($+55\%$) and suppressed AA in the spinal cord (-71%) [26].

To localize the site of action of NE in the brain, alpha-agonist clonidine and alpha-antagonist phentolamine were injected into discrete brain areas in order to observe their effects on EA analgesia [27]. The most impressive results were obtained in the habenula, where clonidine suppressed and phentolamine potentiated the effect of AA. Less marked results were obtained in the PAG and nucleus accumbens, where clonidine lowered the effect of AA, but phentolamine showed no significant potentiation. Injection of the same drugs into the amygdala was without effect in this regard.

ITh injection of phentolamine (alpha blocker) was very effective in antagonizing EA analgesia, as it was in antagonizing the analgesia induced by systemically administered morphine (2 and 4 mg/kg, but not 6 mg/kg, SC) [28]. That EA and morphine may release NE in the spinal cord to exert an analgesic effect was supported by the findings that the spinal content of MHPG, a metabolic end product of NE, was markedly increased after systemic injection of morphine, and that ITh administered phentolamine was effective in blocking analgesia induced by systemically administered, but not ITh administered, morphine [28].

In evaluating the role of GABA in mediating AA, a series of pharmacological tools was used. Systematic administration of 3-mercaptopropionic acid (3-MP), an inhibitor of GABA synthesis and release, markedly potentiated AA. This effect was reversed by aminooxyacetic acid (AOAA), which inhibited GABA transaminase, thus retarding the degradation of GABA. Similar results were obtained when morphine was used instead of EA. Administration of AOAA raised the GABA content in the brain and suppressed EA and morphine analgesia, and this suppression could be reversed by the GABA-antagonist bicuculline, or GABA synthesis-inhibitor isoniazid [29, 30]. In line with these results is the finding that EA and morphine analgesia were attenuated by systematic diazepam, an effect totally reversed by picrotoxin [31]. Radioreceptor assay revealed a several-fold increase in the cerebral content of GABA after the inhibition of GABA transaminase by ICV injection of γ-vinyl-GABA (GVG); in the meantime there was a dose-dependent decrease in the effect of EA and morphine analgesia. A negative correlation was found between the cerebral GABA content and the effect of AA ($r = -0.78$, $n = 23$, $P < 0.01$). The time course of the change in the effect of AA formed a mirror image of that of the cerebral content of GABA [32]. Taken together, the results implicate cerebral GABA as a powerful antagonist for EA and morphine analgesia.

To localize its site of action, a microinjection was done into the PAG of (a) 3-MP, 0.4 μmol, to suppress GABA synthesis and release; (b) GVG, 50 nmol, to increase GABA content, and (c) muscimol, 0.25–1 μmol, to stimulate the GABA receptor. Both EA and morphine analgesia were found to be markedly potentiated by intra-PAG injection of 3-MP and suppressed by GVG or muscimol. No such changes were observed when 3-MP was administered ITh to the rat. The results implicate PAG as one of the strategic sites for GABA suppression of EA analgesia [33].

Endogenous Opioids

Naloxone Blockade of Acupuncture Analgesia

Following the first demonstration of blockade of AA in humans [34] and in mice [35] by systemic naloxone, I was the first to show blockade of AA in rabbits by ICV injection of naloxone [36]. In a mapping study naloxone was microinjected bilaterally into discrete brain areas of the rabbit. Four nuclei were found into which microinjection of naloxone (1 μg in each site) blocked the effect of AA by more than 70%: PAG, nucleus accumbens, amygdala, and habenula; unilateral injection showed significantly less effect [37]. These are the same four nuclei for which microinjection of morphine (5–10 μg in each site) produced marked analgesia [38, 39].

Similar experiments were also carried out in rats, but the results were not as clear. ICV injection of naloxone at doses at large as 20–40 μg was not able to block AA [40]. It was only in rats with attenuated 5-HT function (injected with a moderate dose of PCPA, 200 mg/kg, IP) that ICV injection of naloxone produced a significant attenuation of AA [41]. In these experiments, EA stimulation was used with frequency changing automatically from 2 Hz to 15 Hz every 5 s. Later it was found that the reversibility of AA by naloxone depends very much on the frequency of EA being used [42, 43]. Details will be discussed in the following sections.

Endogenous Opioids as Measured by Radioreceptor Assay

Radioreceptor assay revealed a 33% increase in the cerebral content of opioids in rats after 30-min EA stimulation. A positive correlation was found between the effect of AA and the opioid content in the whole brain ($r=0.61$, $n=20$, $P<0.01$) [44], especially in the forebrain ($r=0.74$, $P<0.01$) and the lower brain stem ($r=0.46$, $P<0.05$), but not in the diencephalon [45].

In contrast to the 33% increase in brain opioids, there was an 18% ($P<0.05$) decrease in pituitary opioids [44]. Bilateral adrenalectomy of the rat produced a significant increase both in pituitary opioid content ($+31\%$) and the effect of AA ($+50\%$), whereas dexamethasone produced a decrease both in pituitary opioid content (-37%) and the effect of AA (-54%) [46]. The mechanism by which pituitary opioids mediate AA remains to be elucidated.

The blood level of opioids was measured by radioreceptor assay in a group of healthy volunteers. Manual needling at one point, SJ.8 Sanyangluo (located in the forearm between the radius and ulnar) for 30 min produced a marked increase ($+54\%$, paired t-test $P<0.001$) in blood opioids, and the postacupuncture opioid level was found to be negatively correlated with changes in the pain sensitivity ($r=0.65$, $n=29$, $P<0.01$). In the group without acupuncture, there was a tendency towards a decrease in blood opioids in the same time period of experimentation ($P<0.01$) [47]. The results were statistically highly significant, although the physiological relevance of blood opioids to analgesia is still awaiting clarification.

β-Endorphin

A radioimmunoassay for immunoreactive β-endorphin (β-EP) was established using antiserum prepared in this laboratory with a titer of 1:3000, cross-reactivity with (Met5) enkephalin (ME) and (Leu5) enkephalin (LE) being less than 0.1% [48]. Experiments in rats showed that EA stimulation of 2–15 Hz for 30 min produced a marked increase in ir β-EP content in the whole brain [49]. A positive correlation was found between the effect of AA and the postacupuncture content or ir β-EP [49]. When the brain was dissected into three parts, the telencephalon, diencephalon, and lower brain stem, the best correlation was found in the diencephalon ($r=0.75$, $P<0.001$), followed by the lower brain stem ($r=0.60$, $P<0.001$) and telencephalon ($r=0.42$, $P<0.05$) [50]. This rank order was different from that found by radioreceptor assay for measuring total opioids in the brain [45], implying a differential role played by β-EP and other endogenous opioids such as enkephalins and dynorphins.

11

While the β-endorphinergic pathway has been clearly defined as emanating from the arcuate nucleus of the hypothalamus (ARH) and ending in the PAG and nucleus coeruleus [51], one report shows that most of the ir β-EP found in the PAG has been N-acetylated during axoplasmic transportation in long tracts and therefore does not function physiologically in the area of the PAG [52]. To test this hypothesis, we injected monosodium glutamate into the arcuate nucleus of the hypothalamus of the rat to stimulate the cell body rather than the fiber tracts. A dose-dependent analgesia was observed, which could be completely reversed by naloxone 1 μg injected into the PAG and partially reversed by intra-PAG injection of β-EP-specific antiserum, and to a lesser extent by ME-specific antiserum, but not by LE-specific antiserum [53]. The results suggest that β-EP in the PAG is not only immunologically active but also physiologically active as a pain-modulating peptide. Supporting this is the finding that the effect of AA can be significantly attenuated by β-EP-specific antiserum which is supposed to bind β-EP being released into the synaptic cleft, thus preventing its receptor activation [54].

Enkephalins

Radioimmunoassays for ir ME and LE were established using rabbit antisera prepared in this laboratory [55]. The titer for ME antiserum was 1:6000, and cross-reactivity to LE, β-EP, dynorphin A (dynA), and Met-enkephalin-Arg6-Phe7 (MEAP) was 1.1%, 0.8%, 0.12%, and 0.1%, respectively. The titer for LE antiserum was 1:8000, cross-reactivity to ME, β-EP, and DynA being 3.7%, 0.1%, and 0.05%, respectively.

EA of 2–15 Hz and 3 V was applied on hind leg points St.36 Zusanli and Sp.6 Sanyinjiao for 30 min, which produced a significant increase in the cerebral content of ir ME and LE in the caudate nucleus ($P<0.05$) and hypothalamus ($P<0.05$). No significant changes were noted in the thalamus, brain stem, or spinal cord. When the ir ME or LE content was plotted against the analgesic effect of EA, a positive correlation was found for ME (caudate: $r=0.44$, $P<0.05$; hypothalamus: $r=0.45$, $P<0.05$), but nor for LE. The results suggest that ME in the brain may play a more important role than LE in mediating AA [56].

To compare the analgesic potency of ME and LE in spinal cord, rats were given ITh injections of the two enkephalins to see their effect on the TFL. ME in the range of 200–800 nmol produced a dose-dependent increase in TFL, whereas LE was at least fourfold less effective. Thus, the analgesic effect of 800 nmol of LE ($+44\%$) was comparable to that of 200 nmol of ME ($+61\%$) [57].

Since enkephalins are known to be rapidly degraded by aminopeptidase and dipeptidyl carboxypeptidase ("enkephalinase"), inhibitors of these two enzymes were administered to try to protect enkephalins from rapid degradation. The analgesic effect of ME (100 nmol) was markedly potentiated by an ITh injection of bestatin, an aminopeptidase inhibitor, and this analgesia was totally abolished by the SC injection of naloxone 1 mg/kg, but not 0.1 mg/kg. Again, combined injection of bestatin with LE (200 nmol) produced no significant analgesia [58]. The results are compatible with the notion that ME is a more powerful analgesic agent than LE, at least at the spinal level. Concerning endogenously released enkepha-

12

lins by AA, there are data to show that the effect of AA is markedly potentiated by an ITh injection of the aminopeptidase inhibitor bestatin or the enkephalinase inhibitor thiorphan [57], and this effect of AA could be blocked by ITh injection of ME-specific antiserum, but not LE-specific antiserum [57].

Similar experiments were also performed in rabbits [59]. A dose-dependent increase in the pain threshold was obtained when bestatin (0.15–0.16 µmol) or thiorphan (0.1–0.4 µmol) was injected ICV. This effect was totally abolished by naloxone (0.125 mg/kg, SC), which strongly indicates that the analgesia is opioid in nature. ICV injection of bestatin or thiorphan in the rabbit was also shown to potentiate and prolong the effect of AA, as well as the analgesia induced by a small dose of morphine (2 mg/kg).

d-Phenylalanine (DPA) is a putative inhibitor of carboxypeptidase A as suggested by Ehrenpreis [60]. ICV injection of DPA was shown to potentiate AA in rabbits [61], rats [62], and mice [9]. This effect was drastically reversed by ICV injection of naloxone [61]. It was interesting to note that while DPA (250 mg/kg, IP) showed little influence on the ir ME and LE content in naive rats, it did produce a marked increase in the cerebral content of ME and LE in rats receiving EA stimulation [62]. In light of this finding a cocktail of bestatin, thiorphan, and DPA was prepared in an attempt to suppress completely the degradation of enkephalins released from nerve terminals. Combined administration of bestatin and thiorphan, 50 µg each, produced only a slight increase of ir ME in the hypothalamus, suggesting that the turnover rate of cerebral enkephalins was rather low in a quiescent status. EA for 30 min increased the ME and LE content in the striatum and hypothalamus by 40%. However, in rats given an ICV injection of bestatin and thiorphan together with an IP injection of DPA, EA increased the ME and LE levels in the striatum and hypothalamus as much as 120%. The results were interpreted to mean that EA accelerated both the production and release of enkephalins, and that the increase in release was compensated and even overcompensated by the accelerated production. Moreover, an increase in the cerebral level of enkephalins induced by peptidase inhibitors was accompanied by an augmentation of the effect of AA, which suggests that these accumulated enkephalins seem to be physiologically active in terms of antinociception [63]. Further studies along this line may lead to a useful in vivo technique for measuring the turnover rate of enkephalins.

Dynorphins

Following the discoveries of enkephalins by Hughes et al. and of β-EP by Li et al. Goldstein and coworkers characterized a new C terminal-extended LE-dynorphin-(1–13) [64], the full sequence of which was later shown to be composed of 17 amino acids and designated as dynorphin A (dynA) [65]. Being 700 times more potent than LE in the guinea pig ileum assay, dynA showed little or no analgesic effect upon IC injection. Thanks to Dr. Avram Goldstein's generous gift of a sample of dynA, dynA was also tried at the spinal level to see whether it produces any analgesic effect. A dose-dependent increase in TFL was found after ITh injection of dynA in the range 5–40 µg (2.3–18.6 nmol). This finding was reported verbally at the 1982 International Narcotic Research Conference held near Boston [66]. The presentation raised a very interesting discussion, because people in many laboratories had tried ITh injection of dynA in rats and failed to see any increase of the nociceptive threshold. The difference between this experiment and that of others seems to be the length of the time period between ITh cannulation and drug administration. A clear-cut result could be obtained only when the injection was performed within 24-48 h of cannula implantation. The decrease in the effectiveness of dynA with time after cannulation was verified later by Herz and coworkers [67] and many others [68]. It is interesting to mention that next to my presentation in the same conference was the report given by M. F. Piercy, who used freehand injection of dyn-(1-13) into the spinal cord of mice and found a marked analgesic effect [69].

The mechanism by which the analgesic effect of dynA fades with time from cannulation has not been fully clarified. Trauma to the spinal cord was shown to increase ir dynA content in the cord tissue [70]. A tentative explanation is that cannulation may cause trauma to the spinal cord and that prolonged and profound release of dynA may lead to a decreased sensitivity of or tolerance to this peptide.

A distinct characteristic of dynorphin analgesia is its relative resistance to naloxone blockade. ITh injection of 5 nmol of dynA or 30 nmol of morphine produced an equipotent analgesic effect – an increase in TFL by 100%-150%. Naloxone (25 nmol, ITh) completely abolished the analgesic effect of morphine, an effect lasting for 1 h. However, it produced only a transient (15 min) and incomplete (50%) blockade of the analgesic effect of dynA [71]. A dose of naloxone as high as 10 mg/kg, SC, was necessary for 50% blockade of dynorphin analgesia [72], pointing to the possibility of activation of kappa-opioid receptors. No cross-tolerance was found between morphine and dynA. However, rats with acquired tolerance to dynA did show cross-tolerance to the kappa-agonist ethylketocyclazocine (EKC) [71]. The results are consistent with the notion that dynA produces analgesia in the rat by activating kappa-opioid receptors in the spinal cord.

While a low dose of dynA (2.5 nmol) elicited analgesia without motor disturbance, a high dose (10 nmol or more) produced various degrees of motor paralysis which was naloxone irreversible. This motor effect seemed to be a feature common to many neuropeptides, including nonopioid peptides such as somatostatin (S. Ferri, personal communication). Since motor paralysis may lead to prolongation of TFL, Spampinato and Candeletti used the tail flick and vocalization tests jointly, the latter being irrelevant to spinal motor function. ITh injection of dynA produced a significant increase in the vocalization threshold, thus providing ample evidence for a decrease in nociception [73]. Recently, dynA-(1-13) at a dose of 30 µg [74] and dynA-(1-13) amide at doses up to 400 µg [75] were given ITh to patients with advanced cancer and intractable pain and proved to be a powerful analgesic without any motor disturbance.

Since the effects of antinociception (small dose of dynA) and motor paralysis (large dose) induced by exogenously administered dynA may represent a pharmacological outcome, it is essential to assess whether endogenously released dynA shows any analgesic effect. EA was used as an effective measure of dynorphin-release induction in the CNS. EA at hind leg points produced a marked increase in the pain threshold measured either in the head or in the tail region. ITh injec-

14

tion of dynA-specific antiserum blocks EA analgesia by 77% as measured in the tail region but not on the head. This blocking effect lasts for at least 4 h [76]. In rabbits with acquired tolerance to EA analgesia by long-term EA stimulation, ITh injection of dynA no longer produces an analgesic effect. No analgesia was noted when dynA was injected into the PAG, nor was EA analgesia blocked by antibody injected into the PAG [76]. These results suggest that dynA reduces the nocicept response in the spinal cord and may play an important role in mediating EA analgesia at the spinal level.

Similar observations were performed for dynorphin B (dynB), a peptide derived from the same precursor as dynA. A dose-dependent analgesia following its ITh administration was observed in rats using the tail flick as a nociceptive test. A dose of 20 nmol of dynB produced a comparable level of analgesia to 5 nmol of dynA (increase in TFL by 90%). For the same degree of analgesia, dynB was 25% as potent as dynA, and 50% more potent than morphine on a molar basis. The analgesic effect of this dose of dynB was partially blocked by naloxone 10 mg/kg, but not 1 mg/kg, given SC. The analgesia produced by dynB was unchanged in the morphine-tolerant rat but was significantly decreased in rats tolerant to ethylketocyclazocine (EKC) [77]. These results suggest that dynB, just as dynA, produces analgesia by activation of kappa- rather than mu-opioid receptors in the rat spinal cord.

Although dynA and dynB were supposed to activate the same category (kappa) of opioid receptors, the combined use of subthreshold doses of dynA (1.25 nmol) and dynB (5 nmol) in the rat produced a synergistic effect. Moreover, ITh injection of either dynA antiserum (1:10000, 0.25-4 µl) or dynB antiserum 1:15000, 0.5-2 µl) dose-dependently attenuated EA analgesia in rats. A combined use of subthreshold doses of dynA antiserum (0.25 µl) and dynB antiserum (0.5 µl) caused an 84% decrease in EA analgesia [78]. The results indicate that dynB is capable of potentiating the analgesic effect of dynA at the spinal cord.

Further study was done to explore the interaction between mu and kappa agonists. It was found that a composition of one-eighth the analgesic dose of dynA (1.25 nmol) and one-quarter that of morphine (7.5 nmol) produces an analgesic effect equipotent to a full dose of either drug applied separately [79]. The analgesic effect induced by the dynA and morphine mixture was not accompanied by any motor dysfunction and was easily reversed by a small dose (0.5 mg/kg) of naloxone. The results indicate a synergism between dynorphin and morphine analgesia. In contrast to the situation in the spinal cord, dynA showed an antagonistic effect on morphine analgesia in the brain, the mechanism of which remains to be elucidated [79]. The implication of mutual interaction between different opioids in the mediation of AA will be discussed below.

Microinjection of Antibodies for Studying Functions of Opioid Peptides

As can be seen from the previous description, the conventional method of administering exogenous peptide to the CNS to study its function has the drawback of not being able to differentiate pharmacological effects from physiological ones. More rational approaches of studying the functions of an endogenously released neuropeptide consist of examining the functional deficit resulting from removal of its action – blockade of synthesis, destruction of nerve terminals, occupation of the receptors, etc. However, the current understanding of the metabolic processing of neuropeptides is far less clear than that for classic neurotransmitters such as acetylcholine and monoamines. As far as is currently known, enzymes involved in the processing of precursor protein and inactivation of biologically active peptide products are specific only to a certain peptide bond, rather than to a whole protein or peptide molecule. It is therefore very difficult, if not impossible, to design a specific activator or inhibitor aiming at the biogenesis or degradation of a single peptide. Moreover, to characterize the receptor of a peptide and to design a potent and specific receptor blocker are generally considered time-consuming tasks which can hardly be expected to be accomplished within a period of years. It is an urgent need in neurobiology research to elaborate a new technique for rapid scanning of the physiological functions for a newly characterized neuropeptide.

The administration of specific antibodies against a neuropeptide to certain brain sites where the peptide is known to be released under physiological conditions would result in a neutralization of the released peptide within the synaptic cleft, thus preventing the peptide from receptor activation. The functional changes elicited by antibody microinjection can be tentatively interpreted as the result of removal of the physiological effects of the authentic peptide.

Previous studies have shown that a precursor protein may produce a number of biologically active peptides which may act on one and the same type of receptor. Pre-proenkephalin, for example, is the common precursor for ME, LE, ME-Arg6-Phe7 (MEAP), ME-Arg6-Gly7-Leu8 (MEAGL), and many other C-terminal extended ME, most of which are acting as delta-opioid agonists. On the other hand, dynA, dynB, α- and β-neoendorphin, and many other C-terminal-extended LE are known to be derived from the common presursor pre-prodynorphin and share the common pharmacological profile of kappa-opioid agonists. The administration of a relatively large dose of the opioid antagonist naloxone would block all types of opioid receptors (mu, delta, kappa, etc.), making the differentiation between the effects of various opioid peptides impossible. In contrast, using the antibody microinjection technique it is possible to inactivate selectively the neuropeptide recognized by the antibody, leaving the other peptides intact to act on the receptors, thereby providing a unique opportunity to differentiate the roles played by closely related peptides [80].

The first series of experiments were performed in 1980 in collaboration with Dr. L. Terenius of Uppsala University, Sweden. Protein-A-purified antibodies against ME or β-EP were sent from Uppsala to Beijing Medical University in a blind coded manner for microinjection into the PAG or the subarachnoid space of the spinal cord of the rabbit to see whether the effect of EA analgesia could be blocked. The results show that ME antibodies block the effect of AA at both the PAG and spinal cord [81]; β–EP antibodies were effective only in the PAG, but not at the spinal level [54]. This is in agreement with a rich enkephalinergic innervation and the very few, if any, β-EP-containing fibers in the spinal cord. Subsequent studies performed in my lab revealed that dynA antibodies were effective in blocking AA only after ITh injection, but not in the PAG [76]. These were the first applications of antibody microinjection technique to study the antinociceptive

16

effect of opioid peptides and to show that various opioid peptides play different roles in the CNS in mediating AA.

Further application of the antibody microinjection technique was used to differentiate the effects of closely related opioid peptides. The chemical structures of ME and LE are very similar, differing only in the C-terminal residue which is methionine in one case and leucine in the other. In vivo studies revealed that ME is at least four times more potent than LE in producing an analgesic effect following ITh injection [57]. Results from an antibody microinjection study indicated that EA analgesia in rats could be blocked by ME antiserum, but not by LE antiserum (57]. This is in agreement with another finding that a positive correlation exists between the efficacy of EA analgesia and the cerebral content of ir ME, but not of ir LE [56], suggesting that endogenous ME plays a more important role than LE in mediating analgesia.

The antibody microinjection technique was also used for differentiating the effect of ME from that of MEAP. MEAP is a C-terminal-extended ME with an analgesic potency as high as, if not higher than, that of ME. Since MEAP is known to be degraded into ME by the angiotensin-converting enzyme (ACE), the apparent effect elicited by MEAP may well be an effect produced by ME. To clarify whether MEAP per se has an analgesic effect, captopril was used to inhibit the activity of ACE, thus preventing the conversion of MEAP into ME. Results of experiments showed that the analgesic effect produced by combined administration of MEAP and captopril to the PAG can be blocked by MEAP antiserum, but not ME antiserum [82], which is certainly in favor of the suggestion that MEAP has an analgesic effect of its own in the PAG of the rabbit. Intra-PAG injection of captopril was also shown to potentiate AA, and this effect was reversed by MEAP antiserum injected into the same site [82]. In the spinal cord, MEAP antiserum failed to affect AA [57], indicating that MEAP is not an important mediator for AA at the spinal level.

In doing an antibody microinjection study it is important to choose a suitable substance for control. The easiest way is to use nonimmunized rabbit serum, or to use affinity chromatography for removal of the specific antibody in question, leaving the rest of the IgG remaining in the antiserum. In 1982, I was able to develop a new way of carrying out control experiments in collaboration with V. Hollt of the Max Planck Institute for Psychiatry. They had raised two antisera in rabbits (HO and UA) against human β-EP, each of which recognized human, porcine, bovine, ovine, camel, and rat β-EP, the only difference being that HO recognized rabbit β-EP, but UA did not. The effect of EA analgesia was seriously attenuated by injecting HO into the PAG of the rabbit, while UA was ineffective [83]. This is one of the best controls ever available for this kind of experiment.

By using antibody microinjections it was possible to characterize some novel functions for dynorphin. Thus, ITh injection of dynA antiserum has been shown to block the analgesic effect of morphine injected into the PAG [84], indicating that dynorphin is involved in the descending inhibitory control from the PAG to the spinal cord. ITh injection of neurotensin caused an analgesia which shared the same feature as dynorphin-caused analgesia, that is the analgesic potency decreased dramatically a week after cannula implantation. This phenomenon prompted me to explore whether the effect of neurotensin was mediated by dynorphin. The supposition was substantiated by the findings that the analgesic effect of neurotensin could be prevented by a large dose of naloxone (100 µg, ITh, but not 1 mg/kg, SC) or by ITh injection of dynA-specific IgG, but not ME-specific IgG [85]. The possibility of the involvement of neurotensin in mediating AA in the spinal cord has been considered.

Frequency-Dependent Release of Opioid Peptides

Traditional Chinese acupuncturists claim that acupuncture at one and the same point can produce qualitatively different therapeutic effects when the needle is manipulated in a different manner: fast or slow, strong or mild, etc. The mechanism is obscure. We have tried to explore this mysterious observation by using EA of various parameters to see whether they could produce qualitatively different physiological effects. EA of different frequencies (2, 15, 100 Hz continuous, and 2–15 Hz alternate) was administered to the rat at St. 36 Zusanli and Sp. 6 Sanyinjiao points, and a marked change in TFL was found. While the analgesia produced by low-frequency (2 Hz) EA could be totally abolished by naloxone (1 mg/kg, SC), the effect of high-frequency (100 Hz) EA was completely resistant to naloxone at the dosage being used [42, 86]. Similar results had been reported by Cheng and Pomeranz and were interpreted to mean that high-frequency EA analgesia was mediated by nonopioid mechanisms [87]. Since the discovery of dynorphin as an endogenous kappa-opioid agonist, the use of a small dose of naloxone as a tool for evaluating the participation of endogenous opioids in certain physiological events should be reconsidered. The dosage of naloxone was, therefore, extended over a range from 0.25 to 20 mg/kg, and it was found that 100-Hz EA analgesia was also naloxone reversible when the dose of naloxone was increased to 10–20 mg/kg [42]. The results imply that the effect of high-frequency EA may be mediated by a subtype of opioid receptor which is relatively resistant to naloxone blockade. The kappa-opioid receptor and its endogenous agonist dynorphins are suspected to be the candidates in this context.

More specific opioid blockers were then used. Analgesia produced by 2-Hz but not by 100-Hz EA was blocked by the ITh injection of the delta selective opioid antagonist ICI 174864, whereas the 100-Hz EA effect was preferentially blocked by ITh injection of MR 2266, a kappa selective opioid antagonist [88].

Cross-tolerance studies revealed that in rats receiving 100-Hz EA for 6 h showed a gradual decrease in the analgesic effect, i.e., tolerance to 100-Hz EA analgesia. These rats, however, still responded to 2-Hz EA stimulation. Rats with acquired tolerance to 100-Hz but not to 2-Hz EA showed a cross-tolerance to analgesia produced by ITh administered dynA [88]. An antibody microinjection study demonstrated that ITh injection of ME antibody blocked 2-Hz but not 100-Hz EA analgesia, whereas dynA antibody blocked 100-Hz but not 2-Hz EA analgesia [89].

In a recent study, spinal perfusion was performed in rats. The amounts of ir ME and dynA in the spinal perfusate was measured by radioimmunoassay. It was found that ir ME increased dramatically in rats receiving 2-Hz EA, but not in rats receiving 100-Hz EA. In contrast, the amounts of ir dynA and dynB increased only in the 100-Hz EA group, and not in the 2-Hz EA group [90]. The results suggest that 2-Hz and 100-Hz EA releases ir ME and dynorphins to produce analgesia via delta- and kappa-opioid receptors, respectively.

As for the β-EP system, neonatal administration of monosodium glutamate (MSG) has been used to destroy the arcuate nucleus of the hypothalamus where the β-EP neurons aggregate. In rats receiving MSG, the analgesic effect elicited by 2-Hz and 15-Hz EA decreased by 77% and 52%, respectively ($P<0.01$), whereas the effect of 100-Hz EA remained intact (-3%). Radioimmunoassay revealed a 46% decrease in the cerebral level of β-EP (data to be published).

All together one can conclude that low-frequency EA analgesia depends on the release of β-EP in the brain and ME in the spinal cord, whereas high-frequency EA analgesia is mediated by dynorphins in the spinal cord.

In clinical practice, it is very popular to use EA of alternating frequencies, 2–15 or 2–100 Hz, for example. In this case, both enkephalins (and/or endorphins) as well as dynorphins are being released. What is the interaction between these opioid peptides at the receptor level? An interesting finding is that dynA antagonizes morphine analgesia in the brain and potentiates morphine analgesia in the spinal cord [79]. Further experiments were performed in which compounds were administered in increasing doses to observe their analgesic effect. ITh injection of 100 nmol of ME alone produced no significant increase in TFL. However, when the subthreshold dose of ME was administered in combination with morphine or dynA-(1–13), a marked potentiation of the analgesic effect of the latter two was observed. Similar results were obtained between LE and morphine, or dynA and morphine [91]. While the molecular mechanisms of the phenomena are still awaiting clarification, it certainly has some practical implication in helping the acupuncturist to choose the right frequency for EA treatment. Clinical experience indicates that the best analgesic effect of EA can be obtained when two frequencies (low and high) shift automatically. It fits very well with the synergism between the analgesic effect of ME (released by low-frequency EA) and dynorphin (released by high-frequency EA). It may also explain the experimental results showing that injection of antibody against a single peptide (either ME or dynA) will produce a drastic decrease of the effect of AA.

Interaction Between Serotonin and Opioids

Previous studies have shown that both 5-HT and opioids are involved in the mediation of AA. It would be interesting to find out whether there is a mutual interaction between 5-HT and opioids.

Experimental data show that in rats injected with PCPA or 5,6-dihydroxytryptamine (DHT), a decrease in 5-HT content was accompanied by an increase in opioid content, as assessed by radioreceptor assay. Linear regression indicated that a complete abolition of the 5-HT content would result in a 65% increase in opioid content [92]. Radioimmunoassay revealed that ICV injection of DHT in the rat produced a significant increase of ir β-EP in the diencephalon, brain stem, and telencephalon. No significant changes were seen in the ir ME or ir LE levels [93].

Blockade of the opioid receptors in the brain by ICV injection of naloxone (20 μg) produced a 14% increase ($P < 0.01$) in cerebral 5-HT content and a 16% increase ($P < 0.05$) in the content of hydroxy-indole-acetic acid (5-HIAA), the metabolic end product of 5-HT. The results imply that lowering the activities of endogenous opioids brought about an acceleration in the turnover of central 5-HT [41].

Thus, a functional interrelationship seems to exist between central 5-HT and opioids, i.e., the impairment of function in any one of them will be compensated by an automatic elevation of the other.

To explore the relation between the effect of AA and the cerebral levels of 5-HT and opioids, the effect of EA analgesia was determined in a group of 27 rats, followed by measurement of the two chemical substrates in the whole brain. The results show that rats with high levels of both central 5-HT and opioids following EA stimulation generally exhibited an excellent analgesic effect; those with elevation of either 5-HT or opioids, a moderate analgesic effect; and those with elevation of neither 5-HT nor opioids, a poor effect. The relation between central 5-HT content (% of control, X_1), opioid activity (% of control, X_2), and the effect of AA (% increase in TFL, Y) can be expressed by the regression equation: $Y = 0.64 X_1 + 0.46 X_2 - 75$ ($r = 0.69$, $P < 0.01$) [94].

In order to ascertain the general significance of the equation, the experiment was repeated under conditions of reduced cerebral 5-HT content by a moderate dose of PCPA or DHT. As mentioned above, a reduction of cerebral 5-HT was accompanied by a rise in opioid activity. This trend was even more marked when EA was given to these animals. Correlative analysis demonstrated that in as much as the decrease in cerebral 5-HT had been compensated by a rise in the level of opioids, the rat retained a fairly good AA effect. However, in those rats in which the cerebral opioid activity failed to make up for the loss in 5-HT, the effect of AA was almost completely abolished. The results of observations in a group of 51 rats can be expressed in a regression equation: $Y = 0.61 X_1 + 0.48 X_2 - 62$ ($r = 0.60$, $P < 0.01$) [92]. The consistency of the general equation under different experimental conditions may well indicate the existence of a substantial interrelationship between cerebral 5-HT and opioids with regard to the effect of AA.

From these results it is obvious that simultaneous removal of the function of both the 5-HT and endogenous opioid systems would result in a dramatic decrease or even complete abolition of the effect of AA [41, 95].

Interaction Between Substance P and Enkephalins

In an experiment in rabbits it was found that intra-PAG injection of substance P (SP) produces analgesia and that the effective sites for this coincide topographically with those of morphine. Moreover, the analgesia produced by focal administration of SP could be blocked by naloxone or enkephalin antiserum, but not by β-EP antiserum administered to the same sites [96]. The results strongly suggest that the analgesia induced by SP is mediated, at least in part, by enkephalins released by short-axoned interneurons located within the PAG. Similar results were obtained in the nucleus accumbens [97] and habenula [98], indicating that SP is a powerful releaser of ME to produce analgesic effects. These results are compatible with those reported by Naranjo et al., who found that analgesia elicited by ICV injection of SP in mice could be antagonized by enkephalin antibodies administered by the same route [99].

In contrast to the fact that injection of SP antibodies or antigen-binding (Fab) fragments into the PAG decreased the effect of AA, administration of SP IgG or Fab fragments at the spinal level increased the analgesic effect [100]. This is consistent with the finding that injection of SP into the PAG in rabbits increased the pain threshold, whereas ITh injection caused a decrease [101].

The aforementioned results make SP a possible candidate as a mediator of analgesia via the release of ME at the level of the PAG, nucleus accumbens, and habenula. At the spinal level the situation might be different. Even if enkephalins are released by EA and suppress the release of SP as shown in the model suggested by Jensen and Iversen [102], there appears to be a sufficient amount of SP released, which can be inactivated by the antibodies. This leads to the potentiation of the analgesia produced by EA from SP antibodies given ITh.

Acupuncture Tolerance

In the early days of the discovery of endogenous opioids, people were hoping for a new group of analgesics without the drawbacks of morphine, e.g., without tolerance and dependence. These expectations, however, soon vanished since administration of a large amount of synthetic opioid peptides caused tolerance and dependence in a way similar to morphine. If EA releases endogenous opioids to exert an analgesic effect, one would expect that EA analgesia also leads to the development of tolerance, when applied continuously or repeatedly with short intervals.

Acupuncture Tolerance and Its Cross-Tolerance to Morphine

While constructing the animal model for AA in rats, I noticed that repeated application of EA stimulation resulted in a gradual decrease of the analgesic effect [8]. This finding was further characterized in the following experiments [103, 104]. Rats were given EA for 30 min of an intensity which increased from 1 V to 3 V. Such a stimulation was repeated after a 30-min interval. A general decrease of the analgesia was observed, so that in the sixth session the analgesic effect was only 24% of the original one. This situation was tentatively termed tolerance to AA (or EA) or simply, acupuncture (EA) tolerance. This status remained for at least 4 h and then recovered slowly. Only after 24 h was the recovery of the effectiveness of AA complete [104]. When continuous EA was used instead of intermittent stimulations, the development of EA tolerance was accelerated, and recovery retarded accordingly [105]. Similar results were also found in the rabbit [106].

To rule out the possibility that the decrease of the EA effect was due to local tissue damage after prolonged stimulation, the test session of EA stimulation was given via needles inserted in the contralateral leg. The effect of EA again reached a very low level, indicating that a central rather than a peripheral mechanism accounted for this phenomenon.

Along with the development of EA tolerance, there was a parallel, although less marked, attenuation of morphine analgesia. At the end of the sixth session of EA, the effect of morphine analgesia decreased to 39% of the original value, implying the development of cross-tolerance [104].

In another experiment a group of rats was given morphine three times a day for 8 days in doses increasing from 5 mg/kg to 50 mg/kg. The effect of morphine analgesia as tested by a challenging dose of 6 mg/kg decreased gradually to only 12% of the original value on day 8. In the meantime there was a parallel, although less marked, decrease in the effect of EA analgesia, reaching 25% of the original level on day 8. Regression analysis revealed that when the effect of EA approaches zero, the effect of morphine remains at one-quarter its original value, and vice versa [104].

It is important to point out that a bidirectional cross-tolerance can be observed only when the primary tolerance has developed to a sufficient degree. Thus, while an IV drip or morphine for 1 day did not impede EA analgesia in the rabbit, as reported by the research group in the first Shanghai Medical College in 1978, one of the same dose for 2 days elicited a clear-cut cross-tolerance [106]. The general profile of EA tolerance is summarized in a review article which appeared in 1982 [107].

Monoamines and GABA in the Development of EA Tolerance

Since the effect of AA is known to be mediated by monoamines and other classical neurotransmitters, it is reasonable to test whether an impairment of these neurotransmitter systems would serve as the mechanism for the development of EA tolerance.

Partial Reversal of EA Tolerance by 5-HTP. In rats with acquired tolerance to EA analgesia from repeated EA stimulation for 6 h, ICV injection of 200 µg of 5-HTP (the direct precursor of 5-HT) elicited a dramatic increase of EA analgesia [108]. In experiments with rabbits, reversal of EA tolerance was noticed when 5-HTP was injected into the lateral ventricles (200 µg) or nuclei accumbens (10 µg) [109]. It could thus be assumed that a functional deficiency of the central 5-HT system might constitute one of the mechanisms for EA tolerance.

However, direct assay showed that the cerebral level of 5-HT and its metabolic end product 5-HIAA were significantly higher (+12% and +110%, respectively) than the corresponding values in control rats, indicating that the decrease of the EA effect could not be accounted for by the depletion of the central 5-HT level or blockade of its release. A turnover study found a 124% increase in 5-HT synthesis and a 91% increase of release in rats with EA tolerance, which is compatible with the net increase in cerebral 5-HT and 5-HIAA levels [108]. Radioreceptor assay revealed that the maximal binding of cerebral 5-HT receptor protein with [^{3}H]5-HT in EA-tolerant rats was of the same level as the control animals [108].

To summarize, although EA tolerance could be partially reversed by 5-HTP, the development of tolerance cannot be explained by the exhaustion of cerebral 5-HT content, the lowering of 5-HT turnover, or the decrease of 5-HT binding sites, thus leaving the possibility of desensitization of the postsynaptic neuron to 5-HT.

Tolerance to Endogenously Released 5-HT as One of the Mechanisms for EA Tolerance. To test whether or not overwhelming release of 5-HT for many hours during repeated EA stimulation will result in the development of tolerance to 5-HT, rats were given six consecutive injections of 5-HTP (25 mg/kg, IP, q.h.) in an attempt to overload the 5-HT receptors with a large amount of newly synthesized 5-HT. After this treatment, the effectiveness of 5-HT was tested by two assessments: (1) the effect of AA in which central 5-HT plays a cardinal role and (2) the hypothermic effect induced by ICV injection of 5-HT. The results indicated that repeated 5-HTP injections caused a decrease in 5-HT hypothermia and a marked attenuation of AA. Besides, attenuation of 5-HT hypothermia was also found in EA-tolerant rats. Thus, tolerance to endogenously released 5-HT may contribute to the development of EA tolerance [18, 110].

Cerebral NE: Exaggeration of the Antagonistic Effect to EA Analgesia. It was previously mentioned that NE in the brain and spinal cord exhibited differential effects on AA: antagonistic action for cerebral NE and facilitatory action for spinal NE, both via α-adrenoceptors [26]. Repeated EA resulted in an exaggerated release of NE both in the brain and spinal cord. A significant increase ($+97\%$) in the level of 3-methoxy, 4-hydroxy-phenylglycol (MHPG), the metabolic end product of NE, with the NE content remaining intact, implied a marked acceleration of its synthesis and release [111]. A partial but significant reversal of EA tolerance was obtained through IP injection of α-adrenoceptor blocker phentolamine or phenoxybenzamine, but not by the β-blocker propranolol. Phentolamine was also effective through ICV injection, but not after ITh injection. The results suggest that repeated or prolonged EA caused profound release of cerebral NE, resulting in an exaggerated antagonistic effect to AA [111, 112].

Spinal NE: Attenuation of Its Analgesic Effect. ITh injection of NE produced a marked increase in TFL in the control rats. This analgesic effect was significantly decreased in EA-tolerant rats. On the other hand, in rats with acquired tolerance to NE from repeated ITh injections (10 µg of NE every 30 min for 3 h), there was a reduction in the effectiveness of EA analgesia [111, 112]. The bidirectional cross-tolerance between the analgesia elicited by EA and that elicited by ITh NE seems to strengthen the contention that tolerance to endogenously released NE in the spinal cord may constitute one of the mechanisms for EA tolerance.

Central GABA and EA Tolerance. Previous studies have shown that GABA in the CNS exhibits an antagonistic effect on AA. In rats with acquired tolerance to EA from continuous stimulation for 6 h, IP injection of 3-MP or isoniazid, inhibitors of GABA synthesis, produces a marked potentiation of AA. This effect of 3-MP could be reversed by ICV injection of muscimol, the GABA-receptor agonist, or by IP injection of AOAA, the inhibitor of the GABA-degrading enzyme. In another experiment 3-MP was given 30 min prior to EA, which lasted for 6 h. The occurrence of EA tolerance was markedly delayed. The results indicate that overactivation of the central GABA system may play a role in the development of EA tolerance [113].

In searching for the mechanisms of EA tolerance I noticed that the cerebral opioid activity as measured by radioreceptor assay remained significantly higher than the control level [103], and that EA-tolerant rats were also tolerant to morphine [104]. These results suggest that the decreased effect of AA might be a result of tolerance to endogenously released opioids, the production of which was shown to be accelerated conspicuously during EA stimulation [44, 45].

Ungar et al. succeeded in isolating an anti-opiate fraction from the brains of morphine-tolerant rats [114], which encouraged me to explore whether an anti-opiate substrate (AOS) existed in the brain of acupuncture-tolerant rats.

Rats were made tolerant to morphine through an 8-day regime [104] and tolerant to EA by giving continuous EA of 2–15 Hz, 3 V, for 6–8 h [115]. Brain extracts of the control, morphine-tolerant, and EA-tolerant rats were subjected to G-25 chromatography and eluted with 0.05 M pyridine-acetic acid buffer at pH 3.9. The fractions collected behind the sodium peak were assayed for anti-opiate activity. In the mouse vas deferens (MVD) test, the brain extract from morphine- or EA-tolerant rats significantly antagonized the inhibitory effect of morphine on electrically stimulated MVD contraction [115]. ICV injection of the brain extract from EA- or morphine-tolerant rats into naive rats suppressed the analgesia induced by morphine (6 mg/kg, SC) or by EA stimulation (2–15 Hz, increasing intensity from 1 V to 3 V in 30 min) [115].

The anti-opiate activity of the brain extract was also tested in another in vitro system. Puiz et al. reported in 1977 that 10-Hz electrical stimulation to guinea pig ileum (GPI) longitudinal muscle strip produced a release of endogenous opioids which suppressed the contraction of GPI elicited by 0.1-Hz stimulation. This effect of endogenously released opioids which could be antagonized by naloxone administered to the bath, could also be blocked by brain extracts from EA- or morphine-tolerant rats but not by brain extracts from normal control rats [116].

Incubation with pronase destroys the anti-opioid activity, indicating that the substance may be a peptide in nature. The fraction containing anti-opioid activity in the GPI assay was further purified by BioGel P 4 and Sephadex G-25 column filtration, followed by thin layer chromatography and DNS-SDS-polyacrylamide gel electrophoresis. The active principle was shown to be a small peptide containing about 10 amino acids but has not been fully characterized [117].

Anti-Opiate Activity of Cholecystokinin Octapeptide. Itoh et al. [118] and Faris et al. [119] reported that cholecystokinin (CCK-8) was a potent antagonist of opiate analgesia. Their findings have been substantiated and extended in my laboratory.

Central administration of CCK-8 in the rat suppressed the analgesic effect of morphine (5 mg/kg, SC) dose dependently in the range 0.25–4 ng. Calculating from the regression equation the dose needed for 50% reversal (RD_{50}) or morphine analgesia was 1.7 ng for ICV injection and 3.1 ng for ITh injection [120, 121]. Compared with the dose of naloxone (1.2 µg, ICV) needed for 50% blockade of morphine analgesia [115], CCK-8 is almost 1000 times as potent as naloxone on a weight basis, or 3000 times as potent on a molar basis. This effect was of immediate onset and lasted at least 4 h. Administration of unsulfated CCK produced no antagonistic effect.

Parallel observations were made on AA. The analgesic effect of EA (15 Hz, 3 V, 10 min) was markedly suppressed by CCK-8, the RD_{50} being 1.0 ng (ICV) and 1.5 ng (ITh), respectively. Again, unsulfated CCK was without any effect [120, 122]. It is interesting to note that CCK-8 antagonized the analgesic effect of EA, no matter whether 2-, 15-, or 100-Hz stimulation was used [122], suggesting an equal potency in antagonizing mu and kappa agonists [90]. On the other hand, CCK-8 had no antagonistic effect on the analgesia produced by ITh injection of NE or 5-HT, suggesting the specificity of CCK-8 as an opiate antagonist [122].

CCK-8 as a Candidate for Endogenous AOS. In order to assess whether endogenously released CCK-8 plays a role in the development of EA tolerance, CCK-8 antiserum was injected into EA-tolerant rats, and an immediate reversal of the tolerance was found [120, 122]. CCK-8 antiserum was also shown to postpone the development of EA tolerance, if the antiserum was injected ICV or ITh into the rat prior to the EA stimulation [122]. The results suggest that activation of the endogenous CCK system, thus exerting an antagonistic effect on opioid analgesia, and may play an important role in the mechanism of EA tolerance.

Similar observations were made on the possible involvement of CCK-8 in morphine tolerance [123]. Tolerance to morphine analgesia was induced by chronic treatment with morphine (5–30 mg/kg, t.i.d. for 6 days). ICV injection of CCK-8 antiserum reverses tolerance to morphine by 50% ($P < 0.001$). ITh injection of the antiserum produces a similar, although less marked, reversal of morphine tolerance. Rats made tolerant to morphine developed a cross-tolerance to EA analgesia. This cross-tolerance is also reversed by the CCK-8 antiserum by more than 50%. ICV or ITh injection of antiserum per se produces no significant changes in the basal level of the TFL, nor does it affect morphine analgesia in naive rats. The results suggest that prolonged activation of opioid receptors may trigger the CCK system in the CNS to exert a negative feedback control, which may constitute one of the mechanisms for the development of tolerance to opioids.

PAG as a Strategic Site for CCK-8 to Antagonize Opioid Analgesia. In a recent study CCK-8 was injected into the PAG of the rat, and it was found that 0.25 ng was sufficient to produce a 50% blockade of the analgesia produced by systemic morphine (5 mg/kg, SC). The dose needed for intra-PAG injection was only 15% that for ICV injection [120], indicating that PAG is a strategic site for CCK-8 antagonism of opioid analgesia.

It is interesting to mention that while ICV injection of CCK-8 or CCK-8 antiserum produces no significant changes in the baseline TFL and in the effect of morphine analgesia, injection of CCK-8 into the PAG of the rat does cause a decrease in TFL, and intra-PAG injection of CCK antiserum or proglumide, the CCK antagonist, produces a significant increase in TFL as well as a potentiation of morphine analgesia. These results suggest that a tonic release of CCK-8 seems to occur in the PAG, which is important for maintaining the pain sensitivity through a delicate balance with the endogenously released opioids [124].

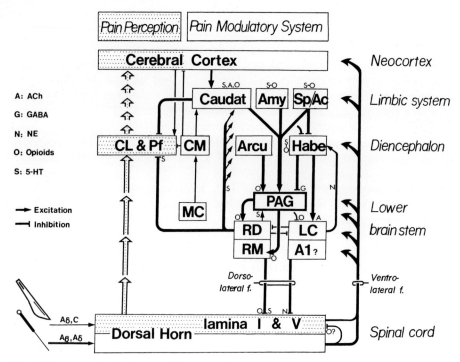

Fig. 1. Diagram showing the possible mechanisms (neural pathways and neurotransmitters) for acupuncture analgesia. For details, see text. *A?*, Perikarya of noradrenergic neurons with descending fibers to the spinal cord (whether it is group A1 or A5-7 remains to be identified); *Ac*, nucleus accumbens; *Amy*, nucleus amygdala *Arcu*, nucleus arcuatus hypothalami; *Caudat*, nucleus caudatus; *CL*, nucleus centrolateralis hypothalami; *CM*, nucleus centromedianus hypothalami; *Habe*, nucleus habenula; *LC*, locus coeruleus; *MC*, nucleus megalocellularis; *PAG*, periaqueductal grey; *Pf*, nucleus parafascicularis; *RD*, nucleus raphe dorsalis; *RM*, nucleus raphe magnus; *Sp*, septum

Summary

In the present review some classical neurotransmitters and some neuropeptides in the CNS for mediating AA have been discussed. Some of them play a facilitatory role, while others are antagonistic. The overall effect of AA thus depends on a dynamic balance between the opposing factors at different levels of the CNS. Various neuronal pathways in the CNS are involved in transmitting the signals triggered by the acupuncture stimulation and in activating the endogenous analgesia system for suppressing nociceptive pathways (Fig. 1). A descending inhibitory control from the PAG to the spinal cord dorsal horn neurons has already been well-defined [125]. Recently, a neuronal circuitry in the brain has been characterized which is very important for mediating AA and morphine analgesia. It is a neuronal loop involving the PAG, nucleus accumbens, amygdala, and habenula, as well as the arcuate nucleus of the hypothalamus. It has been tentatively termed "the meso-limbic loop of analgesia", details of which have been described else-

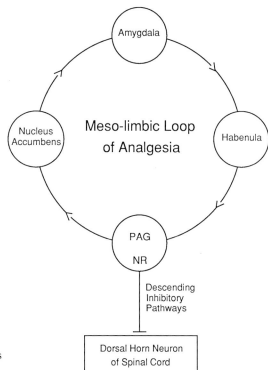

Fig. 2. Meso-limbic loop of analgesia. *PAG*, periaqueductal grey; *NR*, nucleus raphe

where [20, 126–130] and summarized in a review article which will appear in the *Advances in Pain Research and Therapy* series [132] (Fig. 2).

The scope of the present article is limited to the central neurotransmitters in AA. However, the implication of intracellular events such as calcium and cyclic nucleotides in AA and EA tolerance are certainly of great importance. For more detailed information the readers are referred to a monograph published in English covering most of the studies from this laboratory in the field of pain research [131].

References

1. Han JS, Terenius L (1982) Neurochemical basis of acupuncture analgesia. Annu Rev Pharmacol Toxicol 22: 193–220
2. Research Group of Acupuncture Anesthesia, Peking Medical College (1973) Effect of acupuncture on pain threshold of human skin (in Chinese, English abstr.). Chin Med J 3: 151–157
3. Research Group of Acupuncture Anesthesia, Peking Medical College (1974) The role of some neurotransmitters of brain in acupuncture analgesia. Sci Sin [B] 17: 112–130
4. Research Group of Acupuncture Anesthesia, Peking Medical College (1974) Further studies on acupuncture analgesia model in the rabbit (in Chinese). J Beijing Med Coll 1: 18–22
5. Han JS, Zhou ZF, Xuan YT (1983) Acupuncture has an analgesia effect in rabbits. Pain 15: 83–91
6. Research Group of Acupuncture Anesthesia, Peking Medical College (1974) Acupuncture analgesia model in the rat (in Chinese). J Beijing Med Coll 3: 170–173

7. Ren MF, Han JS (1978) An improved tail flick test and its application in the study of acupuncture analgesia (in Chinese, English abstr.). Acta Physiol Sin 30: 204-208
8. Ren MF, Han JS (1979) Rat tail flick acupuncture analgesia model. Chin Med J 92: 576-582
9. Zhang YZ, Tang J, Han JS (1981) Potentiation of electroacupuncture analgesia in mice by intraventricular injection of peptidase inhibitor D-phenylalanine or bacitracin (in Chinese). Kexue Tongbao 26: 1523-1526
10. Fan SG, Xie SZ, Han JS (1987) Afferent fibers transmitting signals for electroacupuncture analgesia as studied by capsaicin. Acupuncture Res (in press)
11. Han JS, Zhang M, Ren MF (1986) The effect of spinal transection on acupuncture analgesia and morphine analgesia. Kexue Tongbao 31: 710-715
12. Huang ZD, Qiu XC, Han JS (1985) The individual variation in acupuncture analgesia: a positive correlation between the effects of electroacupuncture analgesia and morphine analgesia in the rat (in Chinese, English abstr.). Acupuncture Res 10: 115-118
13. Research Group of Acupuncture Anesthesia, Peking Medical College (1975) Effect of p-chlorophenylalanine on acupuncture analgesia in rabbits (in Chinese). Kexue Tongbao 20: 483-485
14. Research Group of Acupuncture Anesthesia, Peking Medical College (1975) Effect of pargyline on acupuncture analgesia in rabbits (in Chinese). Kexue Tongbao 20: 532-534
15. Research Group of Acupuncture Anesthesia, Peking Medical College (1976) Effect of p-chlorophenylalanine and 5-hydroxytryptophan on acupuncture analgesia in rats (in Chinese). J New Med Pharmacol 3: 133-138
16. Han JS, Chou PH, Lu ZC, Yang TH, Lu LH, Ren MF (1979) The role of central 5-hydroxytryptamine in acupuncture analgesia. Sci Sin [B] 22: 91-104
16a. Cheng RS, Pomeranz B (1979) Correlation of genetic differences in endorphin systems with analgesia effects of d-amino acids in mice. Brain Res 177: 583-587
17. Zhao FY, Meng XZ, Yu SD, Ma AH, Dong XY, Han JS (1978) Impacted last molar extraction: effect of clomipramine and pargyline (in Chinese). J Peking Med Coll 2: 79-82
18. Tang J, Li SJ, Han JS (1981) The role of central 5-hydroxytryptamine in acupuncture analgesia and acupuncture tolerance. In: Takagi H, Simon EJ (eds) Advances in endogenous and exogenous opioids. Kodansha, Tokyo, pp 300-302
19. Xuan YT, Zhou ZF, Wu WY, Han JS (1982) Antagonism of acupuncture analgesia and morphine analgesia by cinanserin injected into nucleus accumbens and habenula in the rabbit (in Chinese). J Beijing Med Coll 14: 23-26
20. Xu DY, Zhou ZF, Han JS (1985) Amygdaloid serotonin and endogenous opioid substances (OLS) are important for mediating electroacupuncture analgesia and morphine analgesia in the rabbit (in Chinese, English abstr.). Acta Physiol Sin 37: 162-171
21. Kong BE, Zhou ZF, Han JS (1983) The involvement of serotonergic transmission in periaqueductal grey for electroacupuncture analgesia and morphine analgesia in rabbits. Kexue Tongbao 29: 116-122
22. Li SJ, Han JS (1986) Analgesic effect of serotonin and morphine in spinal cord of the rat (in Chinese, English abstr.). Acta Physiol Sin 38: 19-25
23. Zhang M, Han JS (1985) 5-Hydroxytryptamine in an important mediator for both high and low frequency electroacupuncture analgesia (in Chinese, English abstr.). Acupuncture Res 10: 212-215
24. Han JS, Ren MF, Tang J, Fan SG, Xu JM, Guan XM (1979) The role of central catecholamines in acupuncture analgesia. Chin Med J 92: 793-800
25. Han JS, Guan XM, Shu JM (1979) Study of central norepinephrine turnover rate during acupuncture analgesia in the rat (in Chinese, English abstr.). Acta Physiol Sin 31: 11-19
26. Xie CW, Tang J, Han JS (1981) Central norepinephrine in acupuncture analgesia. Differential effects in brain and spinal cord. In: Takagi H, Simon EJ (eds) Advances in endogenous and exogenous opioids. Kodansha, Tokyo, pp 288-290
27. Zhou ZF, Du MY, Wu WY, Han JS (1981) Effect of intracerebral injection of clonidine or phentolamine on acupuncture analgesia in rabbits (in Chinese, English abstr.). Acta Physiol Sin 33: 1-7
28. Xie CW, Du XL, Tang J, Han JS (1985) Participation of norepinephrine in morphine analgesia in rats (in Chinese, English abstr.). Acta Physiol Sin 37: 258-264

29. Fan SG, Qu XC, Zhe QZ, Han JS (1982) Antagonistic effect on electroacupuncture analgesia and morphine analgesia in the rat. Life Sci 31: 1225–1228
30. Qu ZC, Fan SG, Han JS (1983) Antagonistic effect of cerebral r-aminobutyric acid on electroacupuncture analgesia and morphine analgesia in the rat (in Chinese, English abstr.). Acta Physiol Sin 35: 401–408
31. Fan SG, Wang YH, Du YH, Xu H, Qu ZC, Han JS (1982) Diazepam reduces acupuncture analgesia and morphine analgesia in the rat (in Chinese, English abstr.). J Beijing Med Coll 14: 234–236
32. Zhai QZ, Fan SG, Han JS (1985) The relationship between the changes in GABA content in the brain and the analgesic effect induced by electroacupuncture and morphine. Kexue Tongbao 30: 1543–1546
33. Fan SG, Zhang JY, Qu ZC, Han JS (1984) Involvement of periaqueductal gray in antagonistic effect of GABA on electroacupuncture and morphine analgesia (in Chinese, English abstr.). Acupunct Elektrother Res 9: 122–128
34. Mayer DJ, Price DD, Rafii A (1977) Antagonism of acupuncture analgesia in man by the narcotic antagonist naloxone. Brain Res 121: 368–372
35. Pomeranz B, Chiu D (1976) Naloxone blocks acupuncture analgesia and causes hyperalgesia: endorphin is implicated. Life Sci 19: 1757–1762
36. Research Group of Acupuncture Anesthesia, Peking Medical College (1977) Naloxone blockade of acupuncture analgesia. A preliminary study (in Chinese). Chin J Surg 15: 192
37. Zhou ZF, Du MY, Wu WY, Jian Y, Han JS (1981) Effect of intracerebral microinjection of naloxone on acupuncture and morphine analgesia in the rabbit. Sci Sin 24: 1166–1178
38. Zhou ZF, Xuan YT, Han JS (1984) Analgesic effect of morphine injected into habenula, nucleus accumbens and amygdala of rabbits (in Chinese, English abstr.). Acta Pharmacol Sin 5: 150–153
39. Zhou ZF, Xie GX, Han JS (1985) Substance P produced analgesia by releasing enkephalins in periaqueductal gray of the rabbit. Kexue Tongbao 30: 69–73 (English abstr. in Kexue Tongbao 1983, 28: 1716)
40. Fan SG, Tang J, Chen SL, Han JS (1979) Naloxone blockade of acupuncture analgesia in the rat (in Chinese). Kexue Tongbao 24: 1149–1152
41. Han JS, Tang J, Fan SG, Jen MF, Zhou ZF, Zhang WQ, Liang XN (1980) Central 5-hydroxy-tryptamine, opiate-like substances and acupuncture analgesia. In: Way EL (ed) Endogenous and exogenous opiate agonists and antagonists. Pergamon, New York, pp 395–398
42. Han JS, Ding XZ, Fan SG (1986) The frequency as the cardinal determinant for electracupuncture analgesia to be reversed by opioid antagonists (in Chinese, English abstr.). Acta Physiol Sin 38: 475–482
43. Han JS (1985) Letter to the editor. Pain 21: 307–308
44. Tang J, Han JS (1978) Changes in endogenous morphine-like activity in rat brain and the pituitary gland during electroacupuncture analgesia (in Chinese, English abstr.). J Beijing Med Coll 3: 50–52
45. Zhang WQ, Liang XN, Tang J, Han JS (1979) Effect of electroacupuncture analgesia on endogenous opiate-like activity in discrete brain areas of the rat (in Chinese). Acupunct Anesth 3: 72–75
46. Tang J, Wang Y, Yang SG, Han JS (1981) Pituitary opioids as related to electroacupuncture analgesia in the rat: the effect of adrenalectomy and dexamethocin (in Chinese, English abstr.). J Beijing Med Coll 13: 202–204
47. Xu SL, Fu ZL, Xiang MJ, Lu ZS, Han JS, Tang J, Zhao SL (1980) The effect of manual acupuncture analgesia and its relation to blood levels of endorphin and histamine and the suggestibility (in Chinese, English abstr.). Acupuncture Res 5: 273–281
48. Tang J, Chen CS, Zhou DF, Xie CW, Wang YX, Han JS (1981) Radioimmunoassay for B-endorphin (in Chinese, English abstr.). J Beijing Med Coll 13: 249–253
49. Chen QS, Zhou DF, Wang YX, Tang J, Han JS (1982) Radioimmunoassay for B-endorphin in the brain and pituitary as related to the effectiveness of acupuncture analgesia in the rat (in Chinese, English abstr.). Acupuncture Res 7: 36–39
50. Chen QS, Xie CW, Tang J, Han JS (1983) The effect of electroacupuncture analgesia on the B-endorphin content in discrete brain areas (in Chinese). Kexue Tongbao 28: 312–315

51. Bloom F, Battenberg E, Rossier J, Ling N, Gullemin R (1978) Neurons containing B-endorphin in rat brain exist separately from those containing enkephalin: immunohistochemical studies. Proc Natl Acad Sci USA 75: 1591-1595

52. Akil H, Watson SJ, Berger PA, Barchas JD (1978) Endorphins, β-lipotropin and ACTH: biochemical, pharmacological and anatomical studies. Adv Biochem Psychopharmacol 18: 125-147

53. Fan SG, Wang YH, Han JS (1984) Analgesia induced by microinjection of monosodium glutamate into arcuate nucleus of hypothalamus (in Chinese, English abstr.). Acta Zool Sin 30: 352-358

54. Xie GX, Zhou ZF, Han JS (1981) Electroacupuncture analgesia in the rabbit was partially blocked by anti-B-endorphin antiserum injected into periaqueductal gray, but not its intrathecal injection (in Chinese, English abstr.). Acupuncture Res 6: 278-280

55. Xie CW, Yuan H, Liu YX, Han JS (1984) Radioimmunoassay for met-enkephalin and leu-enkephalin (in Chinese, English abstr.). J Beijing Med Coll 16: 141-144

56. Xie CW, Zhang WQ, Hong XJ, Han JS (1984) Relation between the content of central met-enkephalin and leu-enkephalin and the analgesic effect of electroacupuncture in rats (in Chinese, English abstr.). Acta Physiol Sin 36: 192-197

57. Fei H, Xie GX, Han JS (1986) Differential effects of met-enkephalin, leu-enkephalin and met-enkephalin-Arg6-Phe7 on antinociception and electroacupuncture analgesia in the spinal cord of the rat (in Chinese, English abstr.). Acta Zool Sin 32: 21-27

58. Zhang M, Xie GX, Han JS, Ren MF (1986) A comparison between the analgesic effect of intrathecal injection of methionine and leucine enkephalin (in Chinese, English abstr.). J Beijing Med Univ 18: 19-22

59. Zhou ZF, Jin WQ, Han JS (1984) Potentiation of electroacupuncture analgesia and morphine analgesia by intraventricular injection of thiorphan and bestatin in the rabbit (in Chinese, English abstr.). Acta Physiol Sin 36: 175-182

60. Ehrenpreis S, Balagot C, Comathy J, Myles S (1978) Narcotic reversible analgesia in mice produced by D-phenylalanine and hydrocinnamic acid, inhibitors of carboxypeptidase A. Adv Pain Res Ther 3: 479-488

61. Han JS, Zhang YZ, Zhou ZF, Tang J (1981) Augmentation of acupuncture analgesia by peptidase inhibitor d-phenylalanine in rabbits (in Chinese, English abstr.). Acta Zool Sin 27: 133-137

62. Zhou ZF, Jin WQ, Jan JS (1984) Potentiation of electroacupuncture analgesia and morphine analgesia by intraventricular injection of thiorphan and bestatin in the rabbit (in Chinese, English abstr.). Acta Physiol Sin 36: 175-182

63. Yuan H, Han JS (1985) Electroacupuncture accelerates the biogenesis of central enkephalins in the rat (in Chinese, English abstr.). Acta Physiol Sin 37: 265-273

64. Goldstein A, Tachibana S, Lowney LI, Hunkappiler M, Hood L (1979) Dynorphin-(1-13), an extraordinary potent opioid peptide. Proc Natl Acad Sci USA 76: 6666-6700

65. Goldstein A, Fischli W, Lowney LI, Hunkapiller M, Hood L (1981) Porcine pituitary dynorphin: complete amino acid sequence of the biologically active heptadecapeptide. Proc Natl Acad Sci USA 78: 7219-7223

66. Han JS, Xie CW (1982) Dynorphin: potent analgesic effect in spinal cord of the rat. Life Sci 31: 1781-1783

67. Przewlocki R, Shearman GT, Herz A (1983) Mixed opioid/nonopioid effects of dynorphin and dynorphin-related peptides after their intrathecal injection in rats. Neuropeptides 3: 233-240

68. Herman BH, Goldstein A (1985) Antinociception and paralysis induced by intrathecal dynorphin A. J Pharmacol Exp Ther 232: 27-32

69. Piercy MF, Varner K, Schroeder LA (1982) Analgesic activity of intraspinally administered dynorphin and ethylketocyclazocine. Eur J Pharmacol 80: 283-284

70. Faden AI, Molineaux CJ, Rosenberger JG, Jacobs TP, Cox BM (1985) Increased dynorphin immunoreactivity in spinal cord after traumatic injury. Regul Pept 11: 35-41

71. Han JS, Xie CW (1984) Dynorphin: potent analgesic effect in spinal cord of the rat. Sci Sin [B] 27: 169-177

72. Xie GX, Han JS (1984) Dynorphin: analgesic effect via kappa receptors in spinal cord of rats (in Chinese, English abstr.). Acta Pharmacol Sin 5: 231-234

30

73. Spampinato S, Candeletti S (1985) Characterization of dynorphin-A induced antinociception at spinal level. Eur J Pharmacol 110: 21–30
74. Wen HL, Mehal ZD, Ong BH, Ho WKK, Wen DYK (1985) Intrathecal administration of beta-endorphin and dynorphin-(1–13) for the treatment of intractable pain. Life Sci 37: 1220–1231
75. Han JS, Xie GX, Fei H, Zhang JQ, Yu DS (1986) Dynorphin A (1–13) amide for treating cancer pain. A preliminary report (in Chinese, English abstr.). J Beijing Med Univ 18: 111–112
76. Han JS, Xie GX (1984) Dynorphin: important mediator for electroacupuncture analgesia in the spinal cord of the rabbit. Pain 18: 367–376
77. Han JS, Xie GX, Goldstein A (1984) Analgesia induced by intrathecal injection of dynorphin B in the rat. Life Sci 34: 1573–1579
78. Xie GX, Han JS (1985) The analgesic effect of dynorphin A in spinal cord of the rat is potentiated by dynorphin B. Kexue Tongbao 30: 1688–1692
79. Ren MF, Lu CH, Han JS (1985) Dynorphin-A-(1–13) antagonizes morphine analgesia in the brain and potentiates morphine analgesia in the spinal cord. Peptides 6: 1015–1020
80. Han JS (1984) Antibody microinjection technique as a tool to clarify the role of opioid peptides in acupuncture analgesia. Pain [Suppl] 2: 543
81. Han JS, Xie GX, Zhou ZF, Folkesson R, Terenius L (1982) Enkephalin and B-endorphin as mediators of electroacupuncture analgesia in rabbits: an antiserum microinjection study. Adv Biochem Psychopharmacol 33: 369–377
82. Han JS, Fei H, Zhou ZF (1984) Met-enkephalin-Arg6-Phe7 like immunoreactive substances mediate electroacupuncture analgesia in the periaqueductal gray of the rabbit. Brain Res 322: 289–296
83. Xie GX, Han JS, Hollt V (1983) Electroacupuncture analgesia blocked by microinjection of anti-beta-endorphin antiserum into periaqueductal gray of the rabbit. Int J Neurosci 18: 287–292
84. Xie GX, Xu H, Han JS (1984) Involvement of spinal met-enkephalin and dynorphin in descending morphine analgesia (in Chinese, English abstr.). Acta Physiol Sin 36: 457–463
85. Han SP, Xie GX, Han JS (1987) Involvement of dynorphin in the antinociception induced by intrathecal injection of neurotensin in the rat (in Chinese, English abstr.). Acta Physiol Sin 39: 19–25
86. Han JS, Xie GX, Ding XZ, Fan SG (1984) High and low frequency electroacupuncture analgesia are mediated by different opioid peptides. Pain [Suppl] 2: 543
87. Cheng RSS, Pomeranz B (1979) Electroacupuncture analgesia could be mediated by at least two pain relieving mechanisms: endorphin and non-endorphin systems. Life Sci 25: 1957–1962
88. Fei H, Sun SL, Han JS (1987) New evidence showing differential release from spinal cord of enkephalin and dynorphin by low and high frequency electroacupuncture stimulation. Kexue Tongbao (In press)
89. Xie GX, Han JS (1985) Analgesia produced by electroacupuncture of different frequencies is mediated by different opioids (in Chinese). Kexue Tongbao 30: 388–391
90. Fei H, Xie GX, Han JS (1987) Low and high frequency electroacupuncture stimulations release met-enkephalin and dynorphin A in rat spinal cord. Kexue Tongbao 32: 73–78
91. Huang L, Ren MF, Han JS (1987) Mutual potentiation of the analgesic effects of enkephalin, dynorphin A-(1–13) and morphine in the spinal cord of the rat (in Chinese, English abstr.). Acta Physiol Sin (In press)
92. Han JS, Tang J, Fan SG, Zhang WQ, Zhai QZ (1978) Dual control of electroacupuncture analgesia in rats by central 5-hydroxytryptamine and morphine-like substances (in Chinese, English abstr.). Chin Med J [Engl] 12: 721–725
93. Li SJ, Zhang WQ, Han JS (1984) Increased B-endorphin content in the rat brain following intracerebroventricular injection of 5,6-dihydroxytryptamine (in Chinese). Kexue Tongbao 29: 1138–1141
94. Liang XN, Zhang WQ, Tang J, Han JS (1981) Individual variation in acupuncture analgesia and its relation with cerebral content of endogenous opioids and 5-hydroxytryptamine (in Chinese, English abstr.). Chin Med J [Engl] 61: 345–349

95. Zhou ZF, Xuan YT, Han JS (1982) Blockade of acupuncture analgesia by intraventricular injection of naloxone or cinanserin in the rabbit (in Chinese, English abstr.). Acupuncture Res 7: 91–94

96. Zhou ZF, Xie GX, Han JS (1983) Substance P produced analgesia by releasing enkephalins in periaqueductal gray of the rabbit. Kexue Tongbao 28: 1716

97. Jin WQ, Zhou ZF, Han JS (1985) Substance P in nucleus accumbens of the rat mediates acupuncture analgesia. Kexue Tongbao 30: 464–467

98. Zhou ZF, Han JS (1985) Analgesia induced by substance P administered into amygdala and habenula in the rabbit (in Chinese, English abstr.). Physiol Sci 5: 107–110

99. Naranjo JR, Sanchez-Franco F, Garzon J, Del Rio J (1982) Blockade by met-enkephalin antiserum of analgesia induced by substance P in mice, Neuropharmacology 21: 1295–1298

100. Jessel TM, Iversen LL (1977) Opiate analgesics inhibit substance P release from rat trigeminal nucleus. Nature 268: 549–551

101. Xie GX, Zhou ZF, Han JS (1985) Substance P displays opposite effects on electroacupuncture analgesia in the periaqueductal gray matter and spinal cord of the rabbit (in Chinese, English abstr.). Acupuncture Res 10: 125–130

102. Jessel TM, Iversen LL (1977) Opiate analgesics inhibit substance P release from rat trigeminal nucleus. Nature 268: 549–551

103. Tang J, Liang XN, Zhang WQ, Han JS (1979) Acupuncture tolerance and morphine tolerance in the rat (in Chinese, English abstr.). Beijing Med 1: 34–37

104. Han JS, Li SJ, Tang J (1981) Tolerance to acupuncture and its cross tolerance to morphine. Neuropharmacology 20: 593–596

105. Xie CW, Tang J, Han JS (1981) Tolerance to continuous electroacupuncture and its cross tolerance to morphine (in Chinese, English abstr.). Acupuncture Res 6: 270–273

106. Zhou ZF, Xuan YT, Wu WY, Han JS (1982) Tolerance to electroacupuncture and cross tolerance to morphine in rabbits (in Chinese, English abstr.). Acta Physiol Sin 34: 185–190

107. Han JS (1982) Tolerance to electroacupuncture analgesia and its cross tolerance to morphine. Acupuncture Res 7: 163–174

108. Li SJ, Tang J, Han JS (1982) The implication of central serotonin in electroacupuncture tolerance in the rat. Sci Sin [B] 25: 625–629

109. Xuan YT, Zhou ZF, Han JS (1982) Tolerance to electroacupuncture analgesia was reversed by microinjection of 5-hydroxytryptophan into nucleus accumbens in the rabbit. Int J Neurosci 17: 157–161

110. Li SJ, Tang J, Han JS (1982) Tolerance to 5-HT and its implication in electroacupuncture tolerance and morphine tolerance (in Chinese, English abstr.). Acta Pharmacol Sin 3: 159–163

111. Xie CW, Tang J, Han JS (1984) Central norepinephrine and tolerance to electroacupuncture analgesia (in Chinese). Sci Sin B 9: 818–824

112. Han JS, Xie CW, Tang J (1981) Central norepinephrine. Its implication in the development of acupuncture tolerance. In: Takagi H, Simon EJ (eds) Advances in endogenous and exogenous opioids. Kodansha, Tokyo, pp 303–305

113. Fan SG, Pei Q, Han JS (1985) The role of central GABA in electroacupuncture tolerance (in Chinese). Proc Conf Chin Physiol Soc, pp 106–107

114. Ungar G, Ungar AL, Malin DH, Sarantakis D (1977) Brain peptides with opite antagonistic action: their possible role in tolerance and dependence. Psychoneuroendocrinology 2: 1–10

115. Han JS, Tang J, Huang BS, Liang XN, Zhang WQ (1979) Acupuncture tolerance in rats: anti-opiate substrates implicated. Chin Med J [Engl] 92: 625–627

116. Tang J, Du MY, Han JS (1980) Blockade of the effect of endogenous opiate-like substances released from myenteric plexus of guinea pig ileum in vitro by endogenous opiate antagonist (in Chinese, English abstr.). Acta Physiol Sin 32: 328–331

117. Tang J, Hu CX, Li SJ, Du MY, Huang BS, Zhang NH, Han JS (1980) Isolation and putrification of the anti-opiate substances (in Chinese, English abstr.). J Beijing Med Coll 12: 69–70

118. Itoh S, Komisuura G, Maeda Y (1982) Caerulein and CCK suppress B-endorphin-induced analgesia in the rat. Eur J Pharmacol 80: 421–425

119. Faris PL, Komisaruk BR, Watkins LR, Mayer DJ (1983) Evidence for the neuropeptide cholecystokinin as an antagonist of opiate analgesia. Science 219: 310–312

120. Han JS, Ding XZ, Fan SG (1985) Is cholecystokinin octapeptide (CCK-8) a candidate for endogenous anti-opioid substrates? Neuropeptides 5: 399–402

32

121. Ding XZ, Fan SG, Han JS (1985) Blockade of morphine analgesia by intracerebroventricular or subarachnoid injection of CCK in rats (in Chinese, English abstr.). Acta Pharmacol Sin 6: 237–239
122. Han JS, Ding XZ, Fan SG (1986) Cholecystokinin octapeptide (CCK-8): antagonism to electroacupuncture analgesia and a possible role in electroacupuncture tolerance. Pain 27: 101–115
123. Ding XZ, Fan SG, Zhou ZF, Han JS (1986) Reversal of tolerance to morphine analgesia but no potentiation of morphine-induced analgesia by antiserum against cholecystokinin octapeptide. Neuropharmacology 25: 1155–1160
124. Li Y, Han JS (1987) Cholecystokinin octapeptide (CCK-8) antagonizes morphine analgesia in periaqueductal gray (PAG) of the rat. Brain Res (submitted)
125. Fields HL (1984) Brainstem mechanisms of pain modulation. In: Kruger L, Liebskind JC (eds) Neural mechanisms of pain. Raven, New York, pp 241–252
126. Han JS, Xuan YT (1986) A meso-limbic loop of analgesia: I. Activation by morphine of a serotonergic pathway from periaqueductal gray to nucleus accumbens. Int J Neurosci 29: 109–118
127. Xuan YT, Shi YS, Zhou ZF, Han JS (1986) Studies on the meso-limbic loop of antinociception. II. A serotonin-enkephalin interaction in the nucleus accumbens. Neuroscience 19: 403–409
128. Han JS, Yu LC, Shi YS (1986) A meso-limbic loop of analgesia: III. A neuronal pathway from nucleus accumbens to periaqueductal gray. Asia Pac J Pharmacol 1: 17–22
129. Jin WQ, Zhou XF, Han JS (1986) Electroacupuncture and morphine analgesia potentiated by bestatin and thiorphan adminstered to the nucleus accumbens of the rabbit. Brain Res 380: 317–324
130. Han JS (1986) Physiologic and neurochemical basis of acupuncture analgesia. In: Cheng TO (ed) The international textbook of cardiology. Raven, New York, pp 1124–1132
131. Han JS (ed) (1987) The neurochemical basis of pain relief by acupuncture. Medical Sciences Press of China, Beijing
132. Han JS (1987) A mesolimbic neuronal loop of analgesia. In: Tiengo (ed) Advances in pain research and therapy, vol 10. Raven, New York, p 197

Acupuncture Research Related to Pain, Drug Addiction and Nerve Regeneration

Bruce Pomeranz

Departments of Zoology and Physiology
University of Toronto, 25 Harbord Street, Toronto M5S1A, Canada

Introduction

Research in our laboratory on the mechanisms of acupuncture has proceeded along three main lines. First we studied the neurochemical basis of acupuncture analgesia (AA) and since 1976 have published 39 papers on this subject [47].

Second we studied acupuncture treatment of addiction [11].

Third, we have begun to study the ability of acupuncture to promote nerve regeneration and have 3 papers on this topic [21, 30, 41]. As there are numerous reviews of the overall literature both in this volume and in recent papers [15, 17, 22, 28, 31, 47, 48], the present review will deal mainly with research from our own laboratory.

Acupuncture Analgesia and Endorphins

We began our studies on AA in 1974, recording nociceptive responses from single neurons in the lumbar spinal cord corsal horn of anaesthetized cats using micro-electrodes. Cells in lamina 5 were most appropriate for this study as they receive a convergent input from nociceptors and non-nociceptive fibers. If acupuncture could specifically block pain inputs (nociception) while leaving touch (non-noci-ception) unaffected, this would be an excellent model for studying AA. Clinically, it had been observed repeatedly that, during surgery, AA blocked pain sensations but not touch perception. Moreover, if acupuncture produced AA anesthetized cats, this would rule out the placebo effect, which was the prevalent hypothesis at that time [50]. Finally, this spinal cord study could test the other hypothesis of the time, namely the postulate that AA operated via the Gate Control Mechanism [22], with large diameter inputs from acupuncture needling causing presynaptic inhibition of nociceptive small diameter inputs onto lamina 5 of the spinal cord.

What we found was very surprising. Neither hypothesis was supported; neither placebo nor the Gate Mechanism could explain what we observed: after 30 min of acupuncture the nociceptive responses of the lamina 5 cells were markedly suppressed, while the non-nociceptive responses were unaffected. This was clearly a good model for the clinical observations in which patients undergoing surgery reported intact touch with reduced pain perception. Also placebo was obviously not involved as the cats were anesthetized. However, the biggest surprise was the delayed onset of the AA effect; it took 10 min before any supression of lamina 5 cell response occurred, and 30 min before maximum suppression was observed.

Moreover it took up to an hour after removal of the needles for the neuron's nociceptive responses to return. These delays were reminiscent of the clinical observations in which it took 30 min of needling to prepare the patients for surgery, and where analgesia persisted for hours after the operation terminated. These delays in onset and offset were surprising because the Gate theory could not possibly explain them. Presynaptic inhibition, the main feature of the Gate Mechanism, begins within a few msec and has an offset of a few sec.

Another puzzling result, which also mitigated against presynaptic inhibition (and the Gate theory) was the absence of this AA effect in spinalized cats. Presynaptic inhibition works well in spinalized cats, but this AA effect did not [40].

As the data rate was low (one cell per cat, one cat per week) we were slow to publish these puzzling results [33, 40]. In the interval, endorphins were discovered and their presence in the pituitary suggested an explanation for our puzzling results: perhaps pituitary endorphins were mediating the delayed effects of AA. To test this idea required us to repeat all the lamina 5 experiments, and to try to block the AA with systemic naloxone (a powerful endorphin antagonist). As the data rate was low, we also developed a parallel animal model to test the AA-endorphin hypothesis [34]. This involved awake mice where AA was tested by measuring the latency to squeak after applying radiant heat to the nose [34]. Because of the high data rate and robust analgesia produced by acupuncturing the 1st dorsal interosseus muscle, LI. 4, Hegu point (using 4Hz electrical pulses above the threshold for muscle contractions for 20 min) we were able to publish (in 1976) the first paper in the literature showing that naloxone blocked AA, thus implicating endorphins [34]. A second paper followed soon afterward, in 1977, from Mayer's laboratory showing in humans what we had found in mice, that naloxone blocked AA [20].

The high data rate in mice, furthermore, allowed us to do many control experiments in that landmark paper [34]. Thus, in addition to the 10 mice receiving intraperitoneal (i.p.) naloxone, another group of 10 mice received i.p. saline; a third group received acupuncture alone, a fourth group had sham acupuncture (in non acupuncture locations), a fifth group had naloxone alone, a sixth group had saline alone and a seventh group was merely handled to control for stress (this included restraint and repeated testing for analgesia). The results were unequivocal; naloxone completely blocked AA, while saline did not. Acupuncture alone gave AA but sham needling did not. Naloxone alone produced very little hyperalgesia (and not enough to explain reduction of AA by subtraction). Fig. 1a and b shows these results. Note the characteristic time course.

Since these two early naloxone papers there have been 28 studies reporting successful blockade of AA by systematically administered naloxone (47). There have also been 7 studies which failed to block AA by naloxone (these failures will be discussed later in the review). One of these 28 naloxone papers was our own cat spinal cord single cell electrophysiological study, described above, which finally came out in 1979, showing that i.v. naloxone blocked AA effects (33). Fig. 2a and b shows the single cell recording and Fig. 3 the time course of these results.

A few weeks after the first naloxone results were announced in the research news section of Science [19], a letter to the editor in the same journal justifiably criticized the use of naloxone as the sole proof of the acupuncture-endorphin

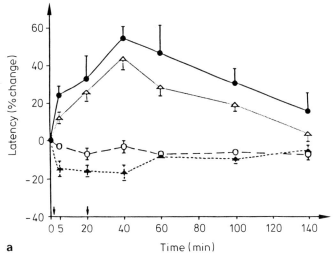

Fig. 1a. Effect of naloxone on acupuncture analgesia. Percentage change in latency to squeak as compared to zero time pretreatment control values. Closed circle solid line for group I – acupuncture; open circle dashed line for group II – sham acupuncture; closed triangles dashed line for group III – acupuncture plus naloxone; open triangles dotted line for group IV – acupuncture plus saline. Each point is average for 10 mice. Bars show S.E. Arrows indicate treatments: for groups I, III and IV acupuncture started after zero time and stopped at 20 minutes; group II received sham needling; groups III and IV received injections at the arrows for zero time and 20 minute boosters

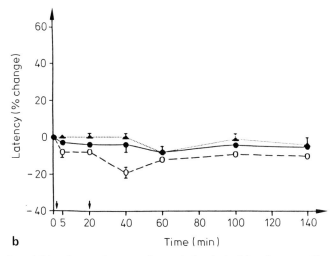

Fig. 1b. Same as figure 1a for additional control groups. Open circles dashed line for group V – naloxone; closed triangles dashed line for group VI – saline; closed circles solid line for group VII – no treatment. At the arrows groups V and VI received injections

A

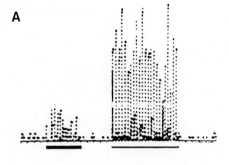

B

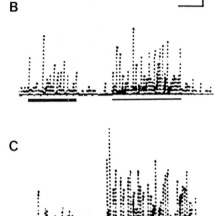

C

Fig. 2a. Records (A to C) from a typical single interneuron in layer 5 of cat spinal cord. The output of an epochal rate meter, bin width 100 msec, is displayed on a storage oscilloscope, each dot representing a single action potential of this cell. As the oscilloscope sweeps from left to right the rate meter produces vertical dots in successively higher positions within bins of 100 msec.
A – Control before acupuncture;
B – 30 min after onset of acupuncture;
C – recovery taken 15 min after needles are removed.
Horizontal bars indicate the duration of the repetitive stimuli: Thick line is light mechanical stimulus, thin line is noxious pinprick. Scale is 5 sec horizontal, 50 spikes/sec vertical

hypothesis [16]. This criticism is based mainly on the argument that naloxone is a drug that might have unknown side effects (unrelated to opiate receptor blocking). Small doses which were effective in reversing AA would tend to implicate receptor effects. But the high potency of naloxone is clearly not enough evidence to prove specificity. However since that letter was written 6 different lines of experimentation have emerged from our laboratory which have independently provided support for the AA-endorphin hypothesis:

1. Four different opiate antagonists block AA.
2. Naloxone has a stereospecific effect.
3. Microinjection of naloxone blocks AA if given into analgesic sites.
4. Mice genetically deficient in opiate receptors show poor AA.
5. AA is enhanced by protecting endorphin from enzyme degradation.
6. AA is suppressed by reducing pituitary endorphins.

38

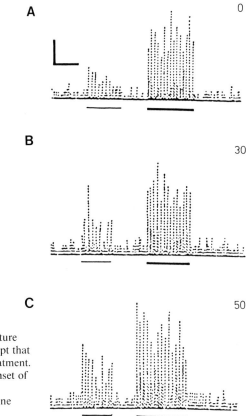

A   0

B   30

C   50

Fig. 2 b. Naloxone reversed electroacupuncture (EA) suppression. Same cell as Fig. 2 a except that naloxone was administered with the EA treatment. *A* - Control before EA. *B* - 30 min after onset of EA and just before needles were removed. *C* - 50 min after onset of EA. Thus, naloxone completely blocked all effects of EA

Details of the 6 lines of evidence supporting the AA-hypothesis are as follows:

1. Using a battery of different endorphin blocking agents, in our mouse squeak paradigm we observed that small doses blocked AA [4]. Thus cyclazocine, or diprenorphine, or naltrexone all blocked AA in the same manner as naloxone. This helps rule out side effects, since it is highly unlikely that all four endorphin antagonists have the same side effects.

2. In the mouse squeak paradigm, we showed that stereospecific receptors are involved in AA [4]. For this experiment, we injected dextronaloxone (an inactive stereoisomer 1000 times weaker than naloxone) and found it to be ineffective at the same doses for which levonaloxone blocked AA. See Fig. 4. Since the most likely side effect of naloxone would be non-receptor membrane fluidization, and because we showed stereospecific naloxone effects which must be receptor mediated, this suggests that endorphin receptors must be involved in AA.

3. In several experiments we showed that intrathecal injections of naloxone (or naltrexone) onto rat spinal cords blocked AA [24, 25]. In one experiment, awake rats with chronic indwelling catheters were given intrathecal naloxone which blocked analgesia from acupuncture-like TENS (they were not given acupunc-

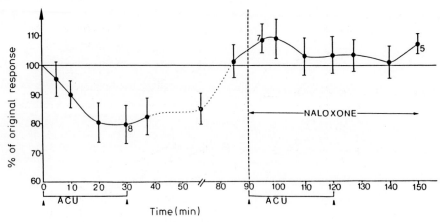

Fig. 3. Naloxone reversed electroacupuncture (EA) supression. EA treatments were given twice: from time zero to 30 min, and again from 90 to 120 min. Naloxone, 0.3 mg/kg i.v., was given at 90 min. Points represent mean of nine cells. Bars show standard error. Percentage of original response for each cell was calculated. Points below the zero baseline denote a decrease in noxious responses. EA alone decreased responses. EA plus naloxone had no effect. Asterisk denotes data for a 20-min interval. The numbers indicate that, occasionally, less than nine cells were averaged into the mean

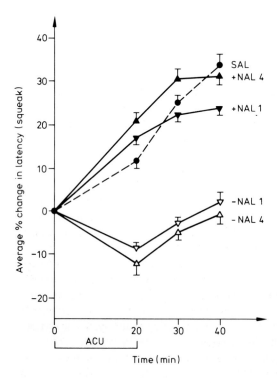

Fig. 4. Effect of (+) naloxone, (−) naloxone or saline on electroacupuncture (EA) analgesia in mice. Ordinate shows percentage change in latency to squeak as compared to zero time pretreatment control value. Positive values denote analgesia. + Nal 1 shows effect of electroacupuncture plus dextronaloxone (1 mg/kg). + Nal 4 shows EA plus dextronaloxone (4 mg/kg). Sal shows EA plus saline (0.9%). − Nal 1 shows levonaloxone (1 mg/kg) plus EA. − Nal 4 shows levonaloxone (4 mg/kg) plus EA. Each point is the mean for 15 mice. Bars show standard error. Arrows indicate time of treatment: EA started after zero time and stopped at 20 minutes; injections were given at zero time and again at 20 minutes (booster). (−) naloxone blocks electroacupuncture analgesia, while saline (0.9%) and (+) naloxone do not

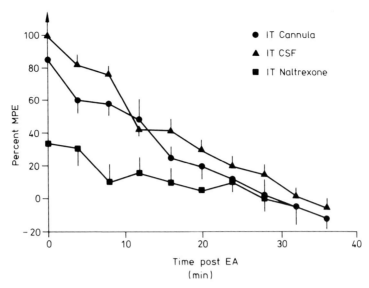

Fig. 5. Effect of EA conditioning stimuli. The changes in latency of tail flick are expressed as percent maximal possible effect, %MPE, plotted against time after cessation of the EA conditioning stimulus. Circles, rats catheterized i.t., no fluid injected (control). Triangles, artificial CSF (15 µl) injected i.t. prior to EA. Diamonds, naltrexone (4 µg) in artificial CSF injected prior to EA conditioning. EA produces a significant increase in tail flick latencies, which is prevented by naltrexone, but not by CSF injection. Vertical lines are S. E. M

ture needles to avoid stressing the rats) [24]. Analgesia was determined by measuring an increase in tail flick latency to radiant heat. In another experiment rats, anesthetized by continuous infusion of pentobarbital, were given intrathecal naltrexone which blocked AA [25]. (See Fig. 5.) In this pentobarbital paradigm acupuncture was given (rather than TENS) as stress was less of a problem under anaesthesia (for example blood pressure was monitored and did not rise during acupuncture treatment).

4. We designed an experiment to test the AA endorphin hypothesis without giving any drugs by use of genetic tools (hence the side effects of naloxone cannot be implicated) [26]. We bred a strain of mice called CXBK, which had previously been shown to respond poorly to morphine because of a congenital deficiency of endorphin receptors. As these mice have about 50% of the usual endorphin receptor activity, they gave less than half the usual AA, proving the need for endorphin receptors (Fig. 6). In another study [43] we showed that these CXBK mice had normal levels of brain endorphins, suggesting that the entire deficiency is located at the receptors. From these genetic studies we speculated that the approximately 30% of humans who do not experience strong AA may have a genetic deficiency in their endorphin system.

5. Even more impressive than blocking AA by naloxone, is enhancement of AA by augmentation of the endorphin system (it is always easier to block than to enhance a biological process). Strong evidence in support of the AA-endorphin hypothesis comes from use of enzyme blockers which protect endorphin pep-

41

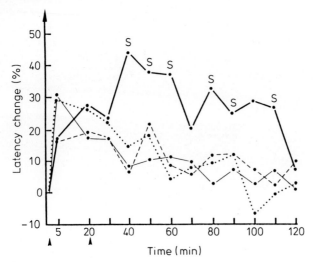

Fig. 6. Analgesia produced by electroacupuncture. Analgesia is expressed as precentage change (from pretreatment control) in latency of hindlimb withdrawal from noxious heat stimulus. Heavy solid line, saline treated C57BL/6By (normal opiate receptor concentration). Light solid line, saline treated CXBK (deficient in opiate receptors). Dashed line, naloxone injected CXBK. Dotted line, naloxone injected C57BL/6By. Electroacupuncture started after zero time and continued for 20 min (arrows). Sampling times showing significant differences between the saline treated groups are designed by 'S'. Each treatment group (each line) represents the average of 15 animals. There was no significant difference in baseline pain thresholds between the two strains (t test, two-tailed, $P > 0.2$). For strain C57BL/6By, threshold was 3.17s (s.d. = 0.83 s); for CXBK this was 3.26 s (s.d. 0.66 s)

tides from degradation. We were the first to show that the D-amino acids D-leucine and D-phenylalamine enhanced AA: we used the mouse squeak paradigm to show this effect [6] (See Fig. 7). That this enhancement was endorphinergic was proved by blocking the enhanced AA by naloxone (i.p.). This D-amino acid effect on AA has since been replicated by Ehrenpreis [12] in humans and by Takeshige in rats [49].

6. We did a series of experiments showing the importance of pituitary endorphins, using the mouse squeak paradigm. In one paper we showed that pituitary removal abolished AA completely [40], while sham surgery did not. In another paper we suppressed beta-endorphin release by injecting the steroid dexamethasone (this worked through the negative feedback effect of steroids on ACTH: since ACTH and beta-endorphin are co-released, dexamethasome injections simultaneously suppressed release of both compounds by negative feedback). Dexamethasone injections 4 h before acupuncture suppressed AA in mice [9]. In a third experiment, we chemically suppressed beta-endorphin in the pituitary by another effective method, that is by feeding mice 2% saline in the drinking water for 3 days; when this was done AA was abolished [9]. Hence these experiments show the involvement of pituitary endorphin in AA.

It is possible that the endorphins released into the circulatory system cannot cross the blood brain barrier in sufficient quantities to cause analgesia. Hence we have postulated that the reverse blood flow in the hypothalamic pituitary portal

42

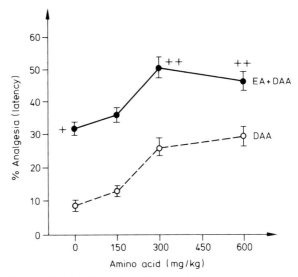

Fig. 7. Dose-response curves of EA + DAA and DAA (D-leucine + D-phenylalanine), in mg/kg. Ordinate shows % of analgesia at 40 min (i.e. % change of average squeak latency at 20 min after EA). Each point is the average of observations on 15 mice. Bars show standard error. Upper curve shows EA + DAA. Lower curve shows DAA alone. At point 0 mg/kg of DAA, saline (0.9%) injection was used. + shows significant EA analgesia ($P<0.01$, t-test, two-tailed). + + indicate EA plus DAA analgesia which is significantly higher than EA plus saline

system can bypass the barriers, and thus deliver endorphins directly to the brain to mediate AA [47].

In addition to these 7 lines of proof of the AA-endorphin hypothesis from our laboratory, there are two experiments from other researchers which also support the AA-endorphin hypothesis:

1. The measurement of endorphin released into the cerebrospinal fluid in humans [46] and animals (see review of Tsou in this volume).
2. The blockade of AA in rats by injection of endorphin antibodies (see review by Han in this volume).

With so much convergent evidence for the AA-endorphin hypothesis, why are there still a few skeptics?

1. Some skeptics [3] note that there are several studies (seven are cited in my recent review) [47], which failed to observe naloxone effects in AA. This is against 28 papers showing naloxone blockade of AA. The reasons for the failed experiments are not always clear. Three of the failed naloxone experiments were observed with high frequency, low intensity stimulation. However, in several animal studies we have found that the AA-endorphin mechanism operates best with low frequency (4 Hz) and high intensity stimulation [5, 25, 32]. In man a similar result was reported [1]. In one of the failed naloxone experiments [3], low

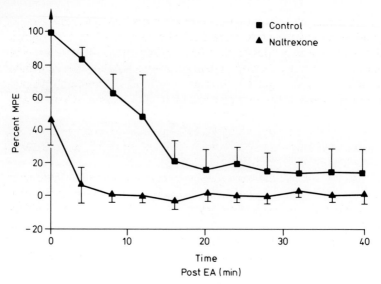

Fig. 8 a. Prevention experiment using i.v. naltrexone. Effects of naltrexone given i.v. before EA treatment began. Triangles show that EA effects were suppressed below the control marked by squares. The curves are significantly different by Manova. Bars show S.E.M. There was prevention

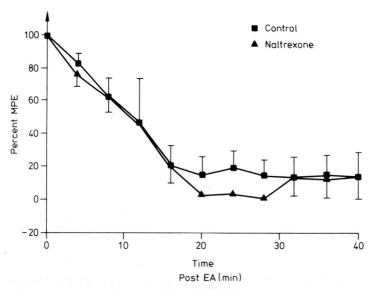

Fig. 8 b. Reversal experiment. Effects of naltrexone given i.v. after completion of EA. The suppression of reflexes by EA (squares) was not affected by naltrexone. There was no reversal

frequency was used; but also low intensity was employed, with an absence of "De Qi" sensations (the deep aching characteristic of strong acupuncture stimulation). The reasons for the three remaining failed naloxone experiments, might be explained by a recently discovered feature of endorphinergic analgesia [32, 39, 51]: Opioid antagonists seem to work best when given before the treatment begins and fail to reverse analgesia that has already been initiated. In other words, naloxone can prevent but often cannot reverse AA (this peculiar naloxone timing phenomenon might be attributed to the poor binding affinity to kappa receptors since several studies implicate dynorphin-kappa effects in AA). (Fig. 8 a and b)

2. Some skeptics state that naloxone antagonism is necessary but not sufficient evidence. We agree, and that is why we did 6 different kinds of experiments to confirm the AA-endorphin hypothesis.

3. Some skeptics attack animal studies of AA as being unrelated to AA in humans. These writers must ignore the numerous experiment in humans which have had the same AA-endorphin outcome as in lower animals. Moreover, the similarity of results across many species proves the generality of these conclusions. Finally if these skeptics are correct, then the entire animal "pain" literature should be discarded, a database which gave us human therapies like endorphins, brain stimulation analgesia, TENS etc.

4. Some skeptics are concerned that AA in animals is merely stress-induced analgesia (which also can release endorphins), and hence is not relevant to AA in humans. The counter-arguments are reviewed elsewhere [29, 47]. For the sake of brevity I will mention two of our experiments: In one study, sham acupuncture in nearby non-acupuncture locations produced no AA while controlling for stress [34]. In another experiment we have studied AA under anesthesia to avoid this problem and obtained similar results as in awake animals [25, 39]. To rule out stress, we recorded arterial blood pressure and found no changes during AA.

In conclusion the overwhelming evidence supports the AA hypothesis. The objections raised by skeptics are easily refuted.

Clinical Applications of AA-Endorphin Effects

Based on these findings Salansky and the author, designed and patented a modified TENS device to activate the AA-endorphin system [38]. Considerable effort was expended to deliver high intensity stimulation to acupuncture points, sufficient to produce "De Qi" sensations for type III muscle afferents without burning and cutting perceptions from type C skin nerves. The success of this new acupuncture-like TENS device is high: in one controlled clinical trial on chronic pain it helped over 90% of cases [8]; in another it helped 75% of patients [13]. Moreover, unlike conventional TENS (using intensities below De Qi levels) the analgesia lasts for many hours, and usually for many days. These TENS machines can be used at home for 30 min a day, on a daily basis to produce cumulative effects [13].

Recent studies in anesthetized rats, show that two successive acupuncture treatments (given for 15 min) 90 min apart cause a potentiation of AA: thus the second analgesia is much more effective than the first [39] (Fig. 9). Moreover, naltrexone (given intrathecally or intravenously) blocks the AA only if given prior to the first acupuncture treatment [39]. This suggests that the first endorphin effect modulates

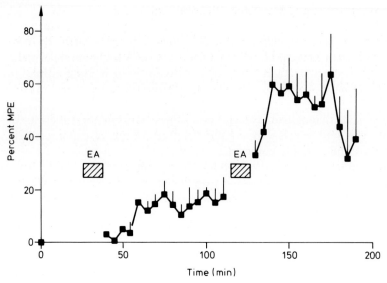

Fig. 9. Effect of EA given twice in succession 90 min apart. Control, no drugs. The first EA produces a small effect which is greatly potentiated the second time. Bars show S.E.M. Mean baseline latency was 3.7 ± 0.1 s (S.E.M.). MPE is maximum possible effect

the synapses so that the second AA (which need not be endorphinergic) is more powerful. This cumulative AA effect of repeated acupuncture treatments has been known for years anecdotally, and has been recently documented clinically [42].

Hence, unlike conventional TENS which must be used continuously because of transient effects, acupuncture (and acupuncture like-TENS) need only be given 30 min a day because of prolonged after-effects, and the cumulative buildup of potentiation from repeated treatments.

Another unexpected result from our new acupuncture-like-TENS device was the permanence of the pain suppression. After 6 weeks of treatment the chronic pain did not return in the 4 to 8 month follow-up period [8]. These apparent "cures" have been often observed with acupuncture, but were previously anecdotal in nature. One possible explanation for prolonged benefit from a limited series of treatments could be that acupuncture releases ACTH along with the pituitary endorphins. In a study in awake horses, we measured elevated blood cortisol after true acupuncture, but observed no change after sham needling [10]. The latter ruled out the possibility that stress was the mediating factor. Perhaps the cortisol produces anti-inflammatory effects in chronic pain due to arthritis, and thus produces "cures". Another possibility is that the cumultive endorphin effects, referred to above, may permanently change the pain circuits.

Acupuncture Analgesia and Other Neuro-Transmitters

Using the mouse squeak paradigm we determined that different frequencies of stimulation caused AA which was mediated by different neurochemicals. As mentioned above, low frequency stimulation (4 Hz) produced AA which was endorphinergic. High frequency stimulation (200 Hz) produced AA which was not affected by pretreatment with naloxone, but was very likely mediated by monoamines (eg. serotonin and/or norepinephrine). For these frequency experiments the needles (in the 1st dorsal interosseus muscle) are electrically stimulated with 0.1 msec biphasic pulses at intensities above threshold to muscle twitch. At 0.2 Hz and at 40 Hz there was no AA. Intervening frequencies were not studied [5]. Cinancerin, a serotonin receptor antagonist was given i.p. and blocked high frequency (200 Hz). PCPA, a serotonin synthesis blocking agent, given i.p. blocked high frequency AA [7]. In contrast, 5 HTP, a serotonin precursor which crosses the blood brain barrier when given i.p., and increases raphe levels of serotonin, enhanced high frequency AA [7]. Yohimbine, an alpha-2 norepinephrine antagonist, when given i.p. blocked 200 Hz AA [7]. Other drugs with less selective effects for serotonin or norepinephrine also produced effects on 200 Hz AA [7]. All together it was apparent that monoamines like serotonin and norepinephrine were involved in high frequency AA [7].

Because i.p. injections could not determine the site of action of the drugs, we changed paradigms to look at the effect of intrathecal injections on high frequency AA in rats. Intrathecal cinancerin had no effects, nor did zimelidine (a drug which potentiates serotonin effects by preventing synaptic uptake). These results suggested that serotonin effects may be due to raphe projections to the forebrain, and not the well known spinal projection. This is a similar conclusion drawn by Han (see Han's chapter). However recent work by Hammond [14] on analgesia in rats produced by brainstem stimulation suggests that descending raphe serotonin mechanisms may work in synergy with descending nonpinephrine pathways. Hence a combined antagonism of both transmitters with two drugs is needed to study this pathway in AA. This has not been tried.

In a recent study of low frequency (4 Hz) AA in anesthetized rats we implicated spinal cord GABA mechanisms. We showed that intrathecal diazepam (Valium), a GABA receptor potentiator, enhanced AA [35]. In addition picrotoxin, a GABA antagonist blocked AA when the drug was given intrathecally [36]. However we did not study high frequency AA and GABA mechanisms.

Acupuncture and Addiction

There have been several clinical studies suggesting that acupuncture can be used to treat the withdrawal symptoms of opiate addiction [52, 44]. In addition one study in rats showed that electroacupuncture of the ear suppressed signs of morphine withdrawal [23]. The same group later showed that this ear acupuncture treatment released endorphins [27], leading to the proposal that acupuncture releases endorphin and thereby overcomes the endorphin deficit caused by negative feedback from exogenous morphine; this in turn overcomes the withdrawal problem.

Hence we undertook a study in mice to determine if acupuncture can overcome the withdrawal signs known to occur in mice addicted to morphine pellets implanted subcutaneously for several days, and in which withdrawal was precipitated by sudden removal of the pellets. Low frequency electroacupuncture was very effective in reducing withdrawal [11]. Moreover, when we studied AA in these mice, we did not observe any cross tolerance; thus, despite tolerance to morphine doses, acupuncture was still effective in producing AA [11].

AA and Afferent Nerve Stimulation

There are two prevalent hypotheses to explain AA. In one, the peripheral nerves are activated (which send messages to the brain to release endorphins etc). In another, energy (or Qi) is supplied, which travels along the meridians to balance the energy flows. To test these hypotheses we did two experiments in the mouse squeak model. In one we injected procaine, a local nerve anesthetic, and found that when nerve impulses were blocked, the AA effect was abolished. In another test, we applied equal amounts of electricity to the acupuncture needles, but used electrical parameters which could not make impulses: no AA was observed in the absence of nerve impulses. In a final experiment, we recorded from the nerves in the brachial plexus of anesthetized mice and determined (from thresholds and conduction velocities) that type II and III muscle afferents were sufficient to elicit AA [37].

Acupuncture and Nerve Regeneration

In the course of numerous lecture tours of the far East, I observed the use of acupuncture in clinics and hospitals (anecdotally) for many conditions other than chronic pain. One of the commonest is the treatment of neurological problems. For example Bell's Palsy, due to seventh nerve injury, has been used in over 100,000 cases in China, with a 90% "success" rate. However as this condition shows spontaneous remissions in over 80% of cases, we would need a controlled clinical trial to determine efficacy of acupuncture compared to sham treatment. This has not been done.

To properly test this phenomenon, we set up a rat model of peripheral nerve regeneration, using lesions to the sciatic nerve in mid-thigh region of adult rats, and treated their legs with electroacupuncture. From the previous literature on electrotherapy of limb regeneration (which has a big component of nerve regeneration) in amphibians [2], we learned that application of a weak direct current (DC) electric field using 1 to 10 μ Amps of current (with the negative pole distal) would have an augmenting effect, so we tried it. We were able to do two kinds of studies after lesioning the sciatic nerve: In one we studied the motorneurons as they regenerated from the mid-thigh to the lumbrical muscles in the foot. In another we observed the growth of a sensory nerve measuring sprouting of the femoral-saphenous cutaneous nerve into the sciatic territory of the foot.

Sciatic Motornerve Regeneration

In this experiment the sciatic nerve was cut in the mid thigh under anesthesia and the two ends resutured to allow the proximal end to grow into the degenerated distal portion. In a control group of rats, the rate of regeneration was determined by reanesthetizing the rats, and measuring the presence (or absence) of electromyograms (EMGs) in the lumbrical muscles of the foot evoked from electrical stimulation of the sciatic nerve via stimulating electrodes proximal to suture site. This was done at different intervals after lesioning (from 25 to 40 days) to determine the "normal" rate of regeneration. As it normally took 35 days for 50% of the lumbrical muscles to become reinervated we decided to do the main study at 30 days after lesioning. During this 30 day interval, different groups of rats received different treatments. One group received electroacupuncture of the denervated paw for 30 min a day, using 10 μAmp DC, with the negative pole distal (the proximal indifferent electrode was placed in the tail to complete the electric circuit). A second group of rats was treated every day with the positive pole of the DC field placed distal to the lesioned sciatic nerve (this would serve as a control as it should not enhance regeneration). A third group received no treatment at all. As predicted from the amphibian limb regeneration studies, only the DC treated group with negative pole distal showed enhanced rates of motor nerve regeneration taking 30 days instead of the usual 35 days [21]. To see whether continuous treatment (24 hours a day instead of 30 min a day) would produce even more enhanced growth rates, we chronically implanted DC batteries in the backs of rats with leads going via wick electrodes into the paw. One group of rats had the DC negative distal and the other had the DC positive distal. This time the motorneurons reached the paw within 25 days of injury, and only in the DC negative group. A third control group had no battery connected, but a wick electrode was implanted. This group did not show as much enhancement as the DC negative group [30].

Sensory Nerve Sprouting

In another series of experiments, the sciatic was severed in the midthigh, but was not permitted to regenerate as it was also tied off with thread. As a result the spared saphenous cutaneous nerve (a sensory nerve which runs parallel to the sciatic from the femoral, and innervates only the medial side of the paw and leg) began to sprout into the lateral paw left vacant by the sciatic nerve lesions. Normally the saphenous nerve can only sprout a few mm to reach the middle of the paw within 21 days after lesion of sciatic. In rats treated for 30 min a day with electroacupuncture (1 μAmp DC), the sprouting was enhanced into the lateral regions of the sciatic territory. Moreover, the DC positive controls failed to show any enhancement [41]. The extent of sprouting was determined in two ways: the extent of anesthesia in sciatic territory as revealed by failure to elicit a flexor withdrawal reflex in the awake rat, and the number of cutaneous nerve fibers stained with a silver stain for light microscope.

Current of Injury

The overall conclusions from these studies were that small DC currents of appropriate polarity (negative pole distal to the growth cone) enhance regeneration of motorneurons, and sprouting of sensory nerves in the leg of adult rats. These results are consistent with previous limb regeneration studies in amphibians, but were now shown for the first time in mammals.

But what does this DC current have in common with acupuncture? Recent evidence from our laboratory [45] indicates that the skin lesion (the hole) created by needling produces a current of injury which persists for 48 hours until the hole heals over. It has been shown [18] that the human skin has a resting potential of from 20 to 100 mv (outside negative). Normally the intact skin has a resistance of 2 to 20 Mohms, while the resistance over an acupunctured site drops to 10 Kohms. This causes the battery (resting potential) to discharge through the hole creating a current of injury of approximately 1 μAmp, negative at the hole [45]. This is the correct current density and polarity to mediate the nerve regeneration described above. We have speculated that the ideal interval beween acupuncture treatments may be every two days because of this 48 hour current of injury caused by needling.

Summary

Studies revealed that acupuncture analgesia is mediated by peripheral nerve stimulation which released endorphins (and cortisol) from the nervous system at high intensity, low frequency stimulation, and monamines at low intensity, high frequency stimulation. Similar parameters were useful in treating morphine withdrawal in mice. However, nerve regeneration was probably enhanced by a different acupuncture effect: the current of injury caused by the hole in the skin.

References

1. Andersson SA (1979) Pain control by sensory stimulation. In: Bonica JJ (ed) Advances in pain research and therapy, vol 3. Raven Press, New York, pp 561–585
2. Borgens RB, Vanable JW, Jaffe LF (1979) Small artificial currents enhances Xenopus limb regeneration. J Exp Zool 207: 217–226
3. Chapman CR, Benedetti C, Colpitts YH, Gerlach R (1983) Naloxone fails to reverse pain thresholds elevated by acupuncture: Acupuncture analgesia reconsidered. Pain 16: 13–31
4. Chèng R, Pomeranz B (1980) Electroacupuncture analgesia is mediated by stereospecific opiate receptors and is reversed by antagonists of Type I receptors. Life Sci 26, 631–638
5. Cheng R, Pomeranz B (1979) Electroacupuncture analgesia could be mediated by at least two pain-relieving mechanisms: endorphin and non-endorphin systems. Life Sci 25, 1957–1962
6. Cheng R, Pomeranz B (1980) A combined treatment with D-amino acids and electroacupuncture produces a greater anesthesia than either treatment alone: naloxone reverses these effects. Pain 8: 231–236
7. Cheng R, Pomeranz B (1981) Monoaminergic mechanisms of electroacupuncture analgesia. Brain Res 215, 77–92
8. Cheng R, Pomeranz B (1987) Electrotherapy of chronic musculoskeletal pain: comparison of electroacupuncture and acupuncture-like transcutaneous nerve stimulation. Clin J Pain 2: 143–149

9. Cheng R, Pomeranz B, Yu G (1979) Dexamethasone partially reduces and 2% saline treatment abolishes electroacupuncture analgesia: these findings implicate pituitary endorphins. Life Sci 24, 1481–1486

10. Cheng R, McKibbin L, Roy B, Pomeranz B (1980) Electroacupuncture elevates blood cortisol levels in naive horses: sham treatment has no effect. Int J Neurosci 10, 95–97

11. Cheng R, Pomeranz B, Yu C (1980) Electroacupuncture treatment of morphine dependent mice reduces signs of withdrawal without showing cross tolerance. Eur J Pharmacol 68, 477–481

12. Ehrenpreis S (1985) Analgesic properties of enkephalinase inhibitors: animal and human studies. Prog Clin Biol Res 192: 363–370

13. Godrey C (1988) Antihabituation, a new TENS modality (submitted)

14. Hammond DL (1985) Pharmacology of central pain modulating networks (biogenic amines and nonopioid analgesics). In: Fields H et al. (eds). Advances in pain research and therapy. Raven Press, New York, pp 499–511

15. Hans JS, Terenius L (1982) Neurochemical basis of acupuncture analgesia. Annu Rev Pharmacol Toxicol 22: 193–220

16. Hayes R, Price DD, Dubner R (1977) Naloxone antagonism as evidence for narcotic mechanisms. Science 196: 600

17. He L (1987) Involvement of endogenous opioid peptides in acupuncture analgesia. Pain 31, 99–122

18. Jaffe J, Barker AT et al. (1982) The glabrous epidermis of cavies contains a powerful battery. Am J Physiol 242: R358–R366

19. Marx JL (1977) Analgesia: how the body inhibits pain perception. Science 196: 471

20. Mayer DJ, Price DD, Raffii A (1977) Antagonism of acupuncture analgesia in man by the narcotic antagonist naloxone. Brain Res 121: 368–372

21. McDevitt L, Fortner P, Pomeranz B (1987) Application of weak electrical field to the hindpaw enhances sciatic motor-nerve regeneration in the adult rat. Brain Res 416: 308–314

22. Melzack R (1984) Acupuncture and related forms of folk medicine. In: Wall PD, Melzack R (eds) Textbook of pain. Churchill Livingston, Edinburgh, pp 691–701

23. Ng LK, Donthitt TC, Thoa NB, Albert CA (1975) Modification of morphine withdrawal syndrome in rats following transauricular electrostimulation. Biol Psychiatry 10: 575–580

24. Peets J, Pomeranz B (1985) Acupuncture-like TENS analgesia is influenced by spinal cord endorphins but not Serotonin: an intrathecal pharmacological study. In: Advances in Pain Research and Therapy, Vol. 9. Editors H Fields et al. Raven Press, N. Y. pp 519–525

25. Peets JM, Pomeranz B (1987) Studies of suppression of nocifensive reflexes using tail flick electromyograms and intrathecal drugs in barbiturate anesthetized rats. Brain Res. 416: 301–307

26. Peets J, Pomeranz B (1978) CXBK mice deficient in opiate receptors show poor electroacupuncture analgesia. Nature 273: 675–676

27. Pert A, Dionne R, Ng L, Bragin E, Moody TW, Pert C (1981) Alterations in rat central nervous system endorphins following transauricular electroacupuncture. Brain Res 224: 83–93

28. Pomeranz BH (1981) Neural Mechanisms of Acupuncture Analgesia. In: Persistent Pain. Editor S Lipton. Academic Press, New York, 241–257

29. Pomeranz BH (1986) Relation of stress-induced analgesia to acupuncture analgesia. Ann NY Acad Sci 467: 444–447

30. Pomeranz BH (1986) Effects of applied DC fields on sensory nerve sprouting and motor nerve regeneration in adult rats. In Ionic Currents in Development. Alan R Liss, Inc, pp 251–260

31. Pomeranz B (1987) Acupuncture neurophysiology. In: Encyclopedia of Neuroscience. Birkhauser Boston.

32. Pomeranz B, Bibic L (1988) Electroacupuncture suppresses a nociceptive reflex: naltrexone prevents but does not reverse this effect. Brain Res 452: 227–231

33. Pomeranz B, Cheng R (1979) Suppression of noxious responses in single neurons of cat spinal cord by electroacupuncture and its reversal by the opiate antagonist naloxone. Exp. Neurol 64: 327–341

34. Pomeranz BH, Chiu D (1976) Naloxone blockade of acupuncture analgesia: endorphin implicated. Life Sci 19: 1757–1762

35. Pomeranz B, Nguyen P (1987) Intrathecal diazepam suppresses nociceptive reflexes and potentiates electroacupuncture effects in pentobarbital rats. Neurosci Lett. 77, 316–320
36. Pomeranz B, Nguyen P. Intrathecal pictroxin potentiates nociceptive reflexes and suppresses electroacupuncture effects in pentobarbital rats. (submitted)
37. Pomeranz B, Paley D (1979) Electroacupuncture hypalgesia is mediated by afferent nerve impulses: an electrophysiological study in mice. Exp. Neurol. 66: 398–402
38. Pomeranz B, Salansky N (1985) Electrotherapy Apparatus and Method. U.S. Patent granted #4-556-064
39. Pomeranz B, Warma N (1988) Electroacupuncture suppression of nociceptive reflex is potentiated by two repeated electroacupuncture treatments: the first opioid effect potentiates a second non-opioid effect. Brain Res. 452: 232–236
40. Pomeranz BH, Cheng R, Law P (1977) Acupuncture reduces electrophysiological and behavioural responses to noxious stimuli: pituitary is implicated. Exp. Neurol 54: 172–178
41. Pomeranz B, Mullen M, Markus H (1984) Effect of applied electric fields on sprouting of intact saphenous nerve in adult rat. Brain Res 303: 331–336
42. Price DD, Raffii A, Watkins LR, Buckingh B (1984) A psychophysical analysis of acupuncture analgesia. Pain 19: 27–42
43. Roy BP, Cheng R, Pomeranz B et al. (1980) Pain threshold and brain endorphin levels in genetically obese ob/ob and opiate receptor deficient CXBK mice. In: Way EL (ed) Exogenous and endogenous opiate agonists and antagonists. Pergamon Press, Elmsford New York, p.297
44. Severson L, Merkoff RA, Chun HH (1977) Heroin detoxification with acupuncture and electrical stimulation. Int J Addict 132: 911–922
45. Shu R, Allan N, Pomeranz B. Electrical resistance measurements of human skin after acupuncture needling (submitted)
46. Sjolund B, Terenius L, Eriksson M (1977) Increased cerebrospinal fluid levels of endorphins after electroacupuncture. Acta Physiol Scand 100: 382–384
47. Stux G, Pomeranz B (1987) Acupuncture Textbook and Atlas. Springer Verlag, Heidelberg, Berlin
48. Stux G, Pomeranz B (1988) Basics of Acupuncture. Springer Verlag, Heidelberg, Berlin
49. Takeshige C (1985) Differentiation between acupuncture and non-acupuncture points by association with an analgesia inhibitory system. Acupunct Electrother Res 10: 195–203
50. Wall PD (1972) An eye on the needle. New Sci, July 20, pp.129–131
51. Watkins LR, Mayer DJ (1982) Organization of endogenous opiate and non-opiate pain control systems. Science 216: 1185–1192
52. Wen HL, Cheng SYC (1973) Treatment of drug addiction by acupuncture and electrical stimulation. Asian J Med 9: 138–141

Mechanism of Acupuncture Analgesia Based on Animal Experiments

Chifuyu Takeshige

Department of Physiology, School of Medicine, Showa University, 1-5-8 Hatanodai, Shinagawaku, Tokyo, Japan 142

Analgesia in response to stimulation of an acupuncture point is produced by two different mechanisms. One is the activation of some of the enodgenous, multiple pain inhibitory systems, and the other is the improvement of the reduced circulation in the painful regions in which possibly the pain causing substance has accumulated.

The present review is focused on the mechanism of acupuncture analgesia (AA) in response to low-frequency electrical stimulation of the acupuncture point as used for surgery, and on AA in response to needle insertion to relieve pain in the muscle.

Acupuncture Analgesia in Response to Low-Frequency Stimulation of the Acupuncture Point

Before the discussion of AA, it is necessary to review briefly the multiple pain inhibitory systems (analgesia-producing systems).

Multiple Pain Inhibitory Systems

In recent decades, several types of analgesia such as opioid and nonopioid, neuronal and neurohumoral, long-lasting post-stimulation and limited during stimulation have been reported. The varying natures of these forms of analgesia were attributed to the numerous endogenous pain inhibitory systems [37, 88]. Activation of a system is dependent upon the peripheral stimulus. When stimulation is by electrical current, different types of analgesic effects are produced at various intensities, frequencies, and stimulation sites through different pain inhibitory systems, since the activated receptor and nerve fiber and their respective connected pain inhibitory systems are different depending on the varying stimulus conditions.

For example, neuronal activities of the dorsal horn, wide dynamic range neurons in response to noxious stimulation are inhibited segmentally by stimulation of non-noxious, low-threshold fibers surrounding or in the proximal area of the noxious stimulation or the contralateral corresponding site [48].

Woolf et al. found that analgesia, as evaluated by the flexor withdrawal response to noxious heating of the tail, was produced by stimulation of the non-

53

noxious afferent in spinal rats. Additionally, strong percutaneous stimulation which excites the $A\delta$ fiber was found to elicit a more powerful analgesic effect than weak stimulation. They further demonstrated that the analgesia is more potent in intact animals than in spinal animals and was naloxone reversible [91, 92].

La Bars et al. reported that when the stimulus strength was increased to a noxious level, the neuronal activities of the wide dynamic neurons in response were inhibited through the descending pain inhibitory system, and they proposed the term "diffuse noxious inhibitory controls" for this pain inhibitory system [35, 36].

It has been reported that low-intensity, high-frequency, transcutaneous nerve stimulation produces a rapidly developing, short-lasting, and segmentally distributed analgesia that is not naloxone reversible. However, high-intensity, low-frequency stimulation induces a long-lasting analgesia with a slow onset that is naloxone reversible [68, 69].

When peripheral stimulation is increased to an electrical stress shock with increasing duration of the stimulation, a different type of analgesia is induced. Stress induced analgesia (SIA), induced by intermittent stress shocks for 30 min (1-s pulse delivered every 5 s), persists long after termination of the stimulation. SIA is naloxone as well as dexamethasone reversible [37] and is blocked by hypophysectomy or adrenalectomy [43]. On the other hand, SIA induced by continuous shock for 3 min (60-Hz sine waves, constant current) is not naloxone reversible when continuous stress shock is applied to the paws but is blocked by naloxone when a stress shock is applied to the front paws [88, 89]. Therefore, a neurohumoral factor is involved in analgesia induced by intermittent stress shock, while continuous SIA is produced by a neuronal mechanism. Opioid and non-opioid mechanisms are involved in neurohumoral as well as neuronal mechanisms [38, 88].

Stimulation for Acupuncture Analgesia Induction

Stimulation of an acupuncture point is necessary to induce AA, while that of a nonacupuncture point does not induce analgesia under the same stimulus conditions. However, different types of analgesia are induced depending upon the intensity and frequency of stimulation of the acupuncture point. Integrated electromyograms of the jaw opening reflex in response to tooth pulp stimulation and of the tail flick response to noxious rat tail stimulation show that they are depressed by the intensity causing the A_β afferent impulse at the acupuncture point, the LI.4 Hegu and St.36 Zusanli points, respectively, without affecting the pain threshold or latency of the noxious response. This depression of electromyogram activity persists long after termination of the stimulation and is naloxone reversible in the LI.4 Hegu point [84], but not in the St.36 Zusanli point [85].

A more intense stimulation, causing muscle contraction around the acupuncture points, is necessary to elevate the pain threshold in the squeak vocalization test [10, 53], the prolongation of tail flick latency [79], and the depression of the writing response with phenylquinone in rats [15, 73].

In human studies, the stimulus intensity for electroacupuncture is generally adusted to a level that is low enough to minimize the production of pain by the stimulus [3, 69]. Such stimulation produces extensive musle twitches. Blocking the skin nerves with a local anesthetic has no effect on AA, but blocking of the muscle nerve abolishes the AA [12].

Low-frequency stimulation is necessary to induce the AA associated with muscle twitch since muscle twitch becomes tetanic contractions in with high-frequency stimulation.

It is thought that AA is produced by afferent impulses associated with muscle twitch since manual needle insertion into the muscle induces AA [46], and low-frequency stimulation initiates the afferent impulses arising from each muscle twitch. A polymodal receptor in the muscle is considered to produce the afferent impulses [25]. In transcutaneous electrical acupuncture point stimulation, an intensity strong enough to cause muscle contraction is necessary to induce analgesia [3].

Analgesia caused by low-frequency stimulation of the acupuncture point develops gradually, reaches a maximum, persists during stimulation, is long-lasting after stimulation termination, and is naloxone reversible [30, 46, 79]. In contrast, analgesia induced by high-frequency, low-intensity stimulation to the acupuncture point develops rapidly and is not naloxone reversible in human studies [68] or in animal experiments [11].

Low-frequency stimulation of the tibial muscle underneath the St.36 Zusanli point or the muscle underneath the LI.4 Hegu point of an intensity sufficient to produce muscle twitch induces analgesia, while analgesia is not induced by the same stimulus conditions applied to the abdominal muscle in rats. Therefore, the tibial muscle stimulation is defined as acupuncture point stimulation, while the abdominal muscle stimulation is defined as a nonacupuncture point stimulation [16, 31, 75].

The stimulus conditions which induce such AA by low-frequency stimulation have been confirmed by evoked potentials in the dorsal part of the periaqueductal central gray (D-PAG): A forcal lesion of the D-PAG abolished AA. Evoked potentials were specifically produced in the D-PAG by stimulation of the acupuncture point, the tibial muscle, and were not produced by stimulation of the nonacupuncture point, the abdominal muscle [20, 74, 75].

The threshold strength to induce muscle contraction of the tibial muscle in rats and the levator auricular muscle in rabbits is coincident with that necessary to produce evoked potential in the D-PAG [20, 54].

In the rabbit experiment, blocking of the skin nerve with local anesthetic did not influence the evoked potentials originating from the muscle contraction. The extent of the acupuncture point was determined by the indication of the D-PAG-evoked potentials. Almost the same potential was evoked in the D-PAG by stimulation on any part of the levator auricular muscle and its nerve [54] (Fig. 1). Therefore, the levator auricular muscle itself was the acupuncture point; similarly, the tibial muscle itself was the acupuncture point of the Zusanli as far as the low-frequency stimulation-produced acupuncture analgesia was concerned. It has been reported by other investigators that stimulation of the upper one-third of the tibial muscle is used for production of AA [39].

The neuronal activities of the reticular formation in response to the noxious tail pinch are inhibited by stimulation of the tibialis anterior muscle, and this inhibition persists after termination of the stimulation [57, 74] (Fig. 2).

55

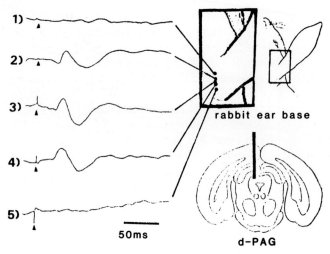

Fig. 1. Potentials in the dorsal part of the periaqueductal central gray *d-PAG; lower right)* evoked by stimulation at the base of the ear lobe *(upper right)*. When sites beyond the auricular levator muscle (*1* and *5; left records*) were stimulated, potentials were not produced, but stimulation within the levator auricular muscle *(2-4)* did evoke potentials [54]

Analgesia induced by such stimulus conditions of the acupuncture point (tibial muscle), as measured by the increase of the tail flick latency [79], vocalization test [53], or writhing response [15, 73], develops gradually, reaches a maximum about 45 min after onser of stimulation, persists long after stimulus termination, and is completely blocked by intraperitoneal (1 mg/kg) naloxone [79] but not by dexamethasone (0.4 mg/kg 24 h before, 0.2 mg/kg given 2 h before) [16].

Pomeranz et al. reported the partial antagonism of dexamethasone on AA in mice [11]. However, dexamethasone had no effect on AA in our experiment in rats [16, 75], while stress-induced analgesia was antagonized by dexamethasone in our lab [86].

The present review concentrates on the analgesia caused by low-frequency stimulation of the muscle corresponding to the acupuncture point [tibial muscle].

Individual Variation in the Effectivenes of Acupuncture Analgesia

Acupuncture point stimulation is not effective in causing analgesia in all animals. Rats have been classified into either acupuncture effective (responder) or noneffective types (nonresponders) using as the criterion a significant increase ($p < 0.05$) of the tail flick latency [78].

Analgesia induced by intraperitoneal (IP) injection of morphine (0.5 mg/kg) is equivalent to AA. Individual variation of morphine analgesia (MA) was highly correlated with that of AA ($r = 0.75$) [78]. AA is abolished by a lesion of the contralateral anterolateral tract (ALT) of the spinal cord, and MA is abolished by a bilateral lesion of the ALT. Analgesia caused by large doses of morphine is reduced but is not abolished by the ALT lesion. The development of AA and MA is depressed by prior intrathecal (ITh) application of naloxone (0.4 µg) [64, 77].

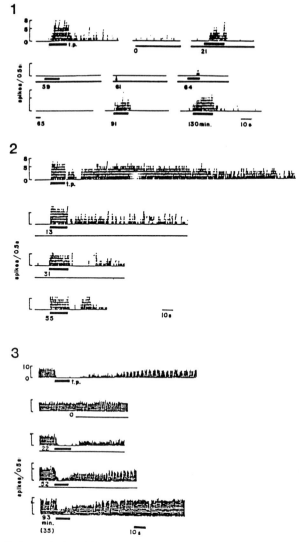

Fig. 2. Three types of neuronal discharge induced in the brainstem by noxious tail pinch and inhibited by stimulation of the acupuncture point: *1*, limited response during pinch; *2*, nonlimited response after start of stimulation; *3*, inhibitory response after start of noxious stimulation. Noxious pinch stimulation indicated by *solid bar*. Acupuncture stimulation indicated by *narrow* bar, and *numbers under bar* indicate time (in minutes) after start of acupuncture stimulation [56]

The equivalent dose of ITh administered morphine to induce AA and MA is 0.05 µg, and analgesia induced by this dose exhibits individual variation in effectiveness parallel to that of AA and MA [64] (Fig. 3).

The dose-reponse relationship between doses of ITh and IP administered morphine and the maximal analgesia is different in responders and nonresponders. This curve was not parallel in the responders and nonresponders and was shifted

57

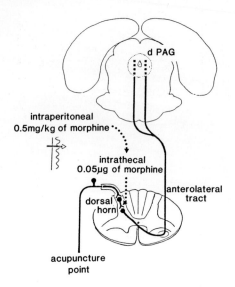

Fig. 3. Morphine analgesia mediated by acupuncture analgesia-producing system

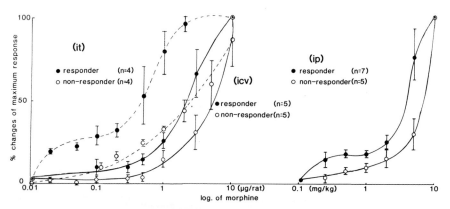

Fig. 4. Dose-response relationships of intrathecal *(it)*, intracerebroventricular *(icv)* and intraperitoneal *(ip)* administrations of morphine in acupuncture responder and nonresponder groups. *Ordinate* shows percentage change in morphine analgesia as measured by tail flick latency. *Abscissa* shows logarithm of morphine dose (μg/rat for intrathecal and intraventricular administration and mg/kg for intraperitoneal administration). *Solid circles,* responder; *open circles,* nonresponder

to the right more for ICV than for ITh [82] (Fig. 4). Analgesia was induced by microinjecting morphine into the nucleus reticularis gigantocellularis (NRGC) which was explored as part of the acupuncture afferent pathway. The dose of morphine required in responders was 0.5 μg, 10 times higher than that given ITh [24]. Hence the most sensitive opiate receptor of the acupuncture afferent pathway must be located in the spinal cord and is activated by IP injected morphine since the ALT lesion abolished this analgesia (0.5 mg/kg). Therefore, the individual variation in the effectiveness of AA as a whole might be determined by that in the spinal cord. After an ALT or D-PAG lesion, the doese-response curve at the low

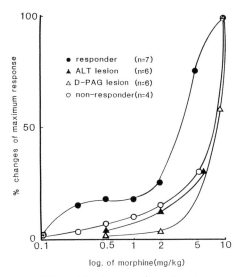

Fig. 5. The effects of lesioning the anterolateral tract (ALT) and the dorsal periaqueductal central gray shown by changes in the dose-response relationship curve of intraperitoneal by injected morphine in responders. *Solid circles,* responder; *open circles,* non-responder; *solid triangles,* after lesioning the bilateral ALT in responders; *open triangles,* after lesioning the unilateral dorsal periaqueductal central gray [82]

doses in responders disappears and that at the high doses becomes similar to that of nonresponders (Fig. 5). Therefore, morphine has at least two actions on the spinal cord. It activates the acupuncture afferent pathway in the responder animals and directly blocks the pain impulses in the spinal cord as reported by Yaksh [93-95]. Willcockson et al. [90] recently reported that the inhibition and excitation of the ALT neuronal activities in response to noxious C-fiber stimulation are induced by morphine microinjection into the dorsal horn, depending upon the application site.

Individual variations of effectiveness are observed in the threshold and magnitude of the D-PAG-evoked potential caused by stimulation of the acupuncture point at the tibial muscle. D-PAG-evoked potentials are blocked by IP injected naloxone 1 mg/kg. The threshold strength necessary to induce D-PAG-evoked potentials is 1 V lower in the responders than in nonresponders, with 0.05-ms rectangular pulse stimulation. The magnitude of the evoked potentials for various stimulus strenghts is consistently about 1.5 times greater in the responders than in the nonresponders, as shown in Fig. 6 [21].

D-Phenylalanine (DPA) is known as an inhibitor of the enkephalin-degrading enzymes (aminopeptidases and carboxydipeptidylpeptidases). After treatment with DPA, the threshold and magnitude of the evoked potentials with D-PAG in nonresponders became similar to that of responders (Fig. 6) [21].

As will be noted later, DPA has an inhibitory action on the analgesia inhibitory system, which inhibits the analgesia-producing pathway connected to nonacupuncture points in the lateral part of the PAG (L-PAG). An L-PAG lesions can eliminate this action of DPA. The close relationship of individual effectiveness

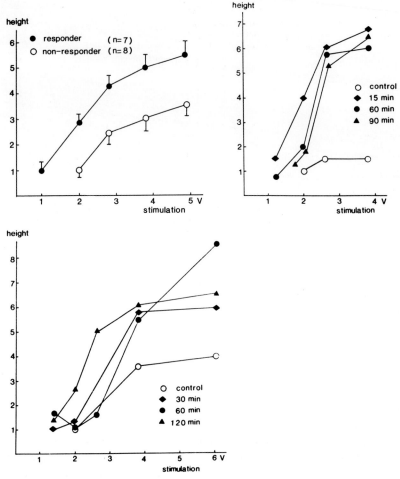

Fig. 6. Comparison of the magnitude of the evoked potentials in the dorsal periqueductal central gray (D-PAG) by acupuncture point (tibial muscle) stimulation between responders and nonresponders, and the effect of D-phenylalanine on these values. *Ordinate* shows the magnitude of potentials evoked in the D-PAG. *Abscissa* shows the stimulus strength (volt) with 0.5-ms duration of rectangular pulse. *Left top:* control; *solid circle,* responder; *open circle,* nonresponder. *Bottom* and *right:* effect of d-phenylalanine (250 mg/kg) on these values in two typical nonresponders; *solid symbols,* after treatment; *open circles,* control [21]

variations of AA and MA does not change following an L-PAG lesion [22]. After DPA treatment, MA and AA in nonresponders become the same as in responders. Likewise, the magnitude of analgesia is the same in responders and in nonresponders following DPA treatment (Fig. 7). Therefore, individual variation in effectiveness is the main feature abolished by DPA.

An individual variation parallel to AA is observed in the stimulation produced analgesia SPA using brain stimulations of all regions pertaining to the acupuncture afferent pathway. Analgesia induction of ICV administered D-Ala-Met-enke-

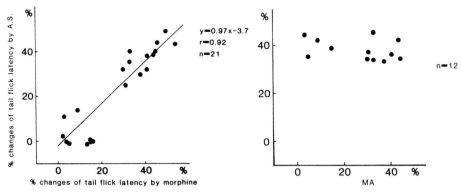

Fig. 7. Relationship of individual variation in effectiveness between acupuncture and morphine (0.5 mg/kg) analgesia after lateral periaqueductal central gray lesioning, and the effects of D-phenylalanine on this relationship. *Left:* acupuncture analgesia 45 min after onset of stimulation versus morphine analgesia 30 min after application. *Right:* morphine analgesia after treatment with D-phenylalanine versus control morphine analgesia [22]

phalin and β-endorphin is augmented by IP administered DPA. However, the most effective sites of DPA action on opioid transmission leading to cessation of individual variation seem to be in the spinal cord since the most morphine-sensitive sites in the acupuncture afferent pathway are located there.

The Afferent and Efferent Pathways Which Induce Acupuncture Analgesia

Since hypophysectomy abolishes caused by low-frequency stimulation of the acupuncture point [10, 30, 53, 58, 73], the pathway from the acupuncture point to the hypophysis is defined as the acupuncture afferent pathway (AAP). AA can also be mediated by activation of the descending pain inhibitory system since lesions on areas of this system abolish AA. This pathway is defined as the acupuncture efferent pathway (AEP).

A lesion on the regions pertaining to both pathways abolishes AA, and analgesia is produced by the focal stimulation of these regions [30, 42]. Potentials are evoked in the AAP regions by stimulation of the acupuncture point [19, 54]. Both pathways have been differentiated by hypophysectomy, since stimulation-produced analgesia (SPA) of the AAP was abolished by hypophysectomy [30], while SPA of the AEP was not [65].

In addition, the nature of SPAs of the AAP and AEP differ. SPA of the AAP is blocked by IP administered naloxone (1 mg/kg), is not blocked by dexamethasone, exhibits individual variation in effectiveness parallel to that of AA, and persists long after termination of stimulation [30]. SPA of AEP is not naloxone reversible, does not exhibit individual variation in effectiveness (a similar analgesia magnitude is observed in all animals), and is short lasting and is limited to the stimulation period [65, 66].

Referring to these properties, the following regions are determined to be part of the AAP: D-PAG, lateral and posterior hypothalamus (LH and PH), lateral sep-

Table 1. Rostral and caudal relationship of the regions in the acupuncture afferent pathway evaluated by the relationship of stimulation-produced analgesia (SPA) and lesioned regions in the acupuncture afferent pathway. SPAs of regions in the vertical column were abolished by lesions to the regions in horizontal row

SPA \ lesion	AH_2	L-SP	CB	D-hip	M-CM	HP	Hypophysis
D-PAG	n=6	n=11	n=7	n=13	n=4	n=8	n=3
L-SP						n=2	
D-Hip						n=5	
MCM				n=5		n=3	
HP	n=3						
AH_2							n=4

n, number of rats [30]; D-PAG, dorsal part of periaqueductal central gray; LH, PH, lateral and posterior hypothalamus; L-SP, lateral septum; D-Hip, dors hippocampus; HP, habenulo-interpeduncular tract; MCM, medial centromedian nucleus; AH_2, anterior hypothalamus.

tum (L-SP), dorsal hippocampus (D-Hip), habenulo-interpeduncular tract (HP), medial centromedian nucleus of the thalamus (MCM), and anterior hypothalamus (AH_2) [30, 42, 56, 75, 77]. Many investigators have reported that analgesia is induced by stimulation of the following regions: PH [62], LH [6, 13, 45], L-SP [1, 9, 18, 45], D-Hip [1], or MCM [47]. The rostral and caudal relationship between these regions has been determined by lesions and SPA of these regions [30]. That is, lesions of the more rostral regions abolished SPA of the more caudal regions, as summarized in Table 1. As illustrated in this table, D-PAG-SPA was abolished by lesions in all other regions and all SPAs, except at AH_2, were abolished by an HP lesion. HP-SPA was abolished by an AH_2 lesion. From these results, the AAP pathway starting from the D-PAG can be seen to diverge into several pathways, converge to the HP, and then reach the AH_2, which is considered as the final region in the AAP, as shown in Fig. 8. Analgesia induced by IP administered morphine (0.5 mg/kg) is similarly blocked by lesions along this pathway [75]. Potentials were evoked bilaterally in these regions by stimulation of the acupuncture point. Since a unilateral lesion was sufficient to abolish AA, a convergent summation effect might be necessary to sufficiently activate these regions in the AAP. It has been reported that the opiate receptors, enkephalin, and β-endorphin are found in these regions [5, 29, 32, 55, 59, 71], although the distribution of enkephalin and β-endorphin is different in the brain [7].

As previously stated, the AAP in the spinal cord is the contralateral-anterolateral tract [64]. In the brainstem, AAP and AEP are within close proximity; therefore both pathways were differentiated by investigating the varying nature of SPA of each and by the individual variation in effectiveness. SPA obtained in nonresponders was limited to the stimulation period and was not naloxone reversible, thus the AEP. However, SPA obtained in responders, persisting long after stimulus termination, was either AAP or a combination of both AEP and AAP. The naloxone reversible part of the analgesia in the combined AAP- and AEP- SPA could be distinguished as SPA of the AAP. From these observations, the reticulogigantocellular nucleus (NRGC) is the AAP in the brainstem (not shown in Fig. 8) [24].

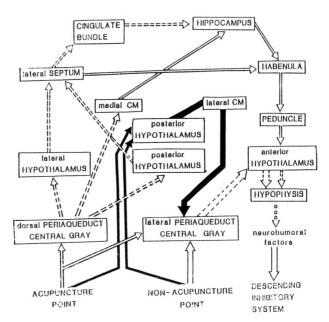

Fig. 8. Central pathways of acupuncture analgesia, nonacupuncture point stimulation-produced analgesia, and the analgesia inhibitory system. *Thin line,* acupuncture analgesia-producing pathway; *thick line,* non acupuncture point stimulation-produced analgesia pathway; *black line,* analgesia inhibitory system [75]

The following regions have been found as AEP: the arcuate nucleus (HARN) [65] and ventral median nucleus (HVM) [66] of the hypothalamus, ventral part of the periaqueductal central gray (V-PAG) [79], raphe magnus (RM) [77], and reticular paragigantocellular nucleus (NRPG) [24, 49]. SPA of the HARN is blocked by an HVM lesion, dopamine antagonist, pimozide, dorsolateral funiculus (DLF) lesion of the spinal cord, and concurrent application of a serotonergic antagonist (methysergide) and a noradrenergic antagonist (phentolamine), but not by naloxone and hypophysectomy [66]. Potentials are evoked in the HVM by stimulation of the HARN. AA is abolished by pimozide [23].

HVM-SPA is partially abolished by a V-PAG lesion [66] and by a NRPG lesion [49]. Potentials are evoked in the V-PAG [66] and NRPG by stimulation of HVM [49]. V-PAG- and RM-SPAs are abolished by methysergide, while NRPG-SPA is abolished by ITh administered phentolamine [49]. AA and D-PAG-SPA are abolished by concurrent lesions of the RM and NRPG and are partially abolished by a V-PAG lesion and by methysergide [79]. AEP-SPA is not blocked by naloxone.

From these results, it can be concluded that the AEP originates at the HARN and descends to the HVM, involving the dopamine neurons [65], and then descends through two pathways. One pathway is the serotonergic pain inhibitory system through the V-PAG and RM, and the other is the noradrenergic pain inhibitory system via the NRPG (Fig. 9) [49, 79]. The neurotransmitters from the HVM to the V-PAG and the NRPG are not yet know (Fig. 9).

63

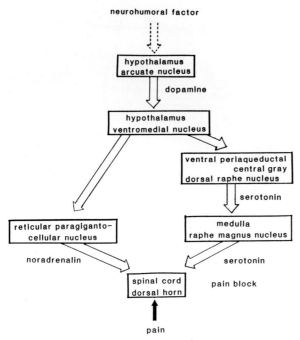

neurohumoral factor

hypothalamus
arcuate nucleus

dopamine

hypothalamus
ventromedial nucleus

ventral periaqueductal
central gray
dorsal raphe nucleus

serotonin

reticular paragiganto-
cellular nucleus

medulla
raphe magnus nucleus

noradrenalin

serotonin

spinal cord
dorsal horn

pain block

pain

Fig. 9. Neuronal connection of the acupuncture efferent pathway (descending pain inhibitory system). The arcuate nucleus is activated by microinjection of morphine. It is connected to the ventromedial nucleus, involving dopaminergic neurons. Two pathways descend from the ventromedial nucleus: one is serotonergic via the ventral periaqueductal central gray and raphe magnus nucleus, the other is noradrenergic via the reticular paragigantocellular nucleus [49, 65, 66]

It was reported that the noradrenergic neuron is not found in the NRPG [60]; therefore, the descending fiber from the NRPG reaches the noradrenergic neurons and inhibits the pain impulse in the spinal cord. It has been reported that analgesia is induced by microinjection of morphine into some regions of the AEP, such as the NRPG [2] and ventrolateral part of the PAG [96]; however, the opiate receptore may not be involved in the AEP producing AA since AEP-SPA is not naloxone reversible.

Analgesia Induced by Stimulation of the Nonacupuncture Point Following Lesioning of the Analgesia Inhibitory System

Analgesia was not induced by stimulation of the abdominal muscle, chosen as a representative of nonacupuncture points (NAP); The NAP was stimulated at the same intensity and frequency as applied to the tibial muscle, the acupuncture point (AP). However, analgesia was induced by stimulation of the abdominal muscle NAP after lesioning the lateral part of the thalamus centromedian nucleus (L-

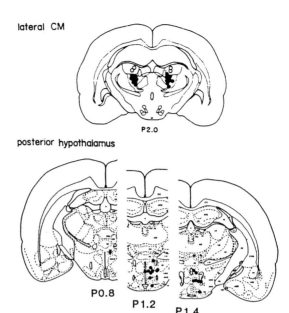

lateral CM

P2.0

posterior hypothalamus

Fig. 10. Localization of the analgesia inhibitory system in the lateral centromedian nucleus of the thalamus *(LCM)* and the posterior hypothalamus [17, 50]. *Blackened areas* show the sites of the lesions

P0.8   P1.2   P1.4

CM) and by lesioning part of the posterior hypothalamus (I-PH) by electrode insertion [17, 31, 50] (Fig. 10). Hence L-CM and I-PH were designated as parts of ad analgesia inhibitory system (AIS) as shown in Fig. 8. Analgesia produced from NAP after lesioning the AIS was called non-acupuncture point analgesia (NAA) and differs from true AA in the following ways: (a) it is blocked by dexamethasone (0.4 mg/kg, 24 h before experiment; 0.2 mg/kg, 2 h before hand), but not by IP administerd naloxone (1 mg/kg), (b) it does not exhibit individual variation in effectiveness, and (c) it is not blocked by lesions of the AAP, but is blocked by lesions of other regions, such as the L-PAG or part of the anterior hypothalamus (AH$_1$) [17, 31, 50], as illustrated in Fig. 11.

Like AA, analgesia induced by stimulation of the NAP is blocked by hypophysectomy, adrenectomy [58], and by lesioning the AEP [65]. Therefore, the AP and NAP are connected to different pathways leading to the hpyophysis, and I-PH and L-CM form part of the AIS for the NAA, and the descending pain inhibitory systems have in common the production of AA and NAA (see Fig. 8).

Analgesia induced by stimulation of the AP and analgesia induced by IP administered morphine (0.5 mg/kg) are augmented by lesioning the AIS [50]. Yeung et al. reported an augmentation in the level of morphine analgesia after lesioning the medial thalamus or PH [97].

Analgesia cessation after lesioning the AAP was reproduced by stimulation of the AP after lesioning the AIS. Recurring analgesia was abolished by lesioning the L-PAG and largely abolished by dexamethasone. The remaining analgesias were blocked by naloxone. L-PAG- and AH$_1$-SPAs were similarly antagonized by dexamethasone and naloxone [31]. Therefore, AP is also connected to the NAP pathway by adding naloxone reversible analgesia as schematically shown in Fig. 12 [31, 86].

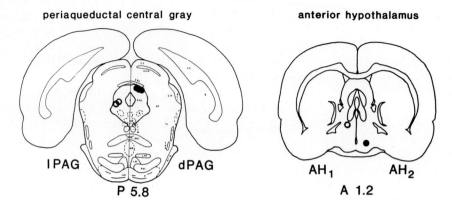

periaqueductal central gray   anterior hypothalamus

l PAG   dPAG   AH$_1$ AH$_2$

P 5.8   A 1.2

Fig. 11. The difference between the acupuncture afferent pathway and nonacupuncture point stimulation-produced analgesia pathway in the periaqueductal central gray *(PAG)* and anterior hypothalamus *(AH)*. The acupuncture afferent pathway in the PAG is located in the dorsal part *(d)* of the PAG *(solid circles),* while the nonacupuncture point stimulation-produced analgesia is located in the lateral part *l; (open circles).* The two pathways are in different locations in the AH$_2$ shown on the *right half* of the slice *(closed circles)* and AH$_1$ *(open circles)* shown on the *left half* of the slice [17, 31, 50]

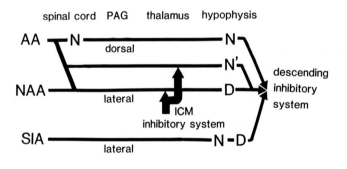

N: naloxone reversal

D: dexamethasone reversal

Fig. 12. Schema of the acupuncture *(AA)* and nonacupuncture point stimulation-produced analgesia *(NAA).* The acupuncture point is connected to the naloxone-reversible, analgesia-producing system *(N)* via the dorsal portion of the periaqueductal central gray *(PAG).* The non-acupuncture point is connected to the dexamethasone-reversible, analgesia-producing system *(D)* through the lateral portion of the PAG. The acupuncture point is also connected to the naloxone-reversible pathway *(N′).* This pathway is inhibited in the lateral PAG by the analgesia inhibitory system, which is activated by stimulation of acupuncture and nonacupuncture points [31]. Stress-induced analgesia (SIA) is produced by naloxone and the dexamethasone-reversible, analgesia-producing pathways *(N-D)* through the L-PAG but is not inhibited by the analgesia inhibitory system [86]

It is possible to stimulate the AIS via a lesioning electrode inserted into it. Augmented analgesia in AA and MA after lesioning the AIS is inhibited by stimulation of the AIS without affecting the original AA or MA during stimulation. The NAA and the recurrent analgesia in AA and MA, after lesioning both the AIS and the AAP, are completely inhibited by stimulation of the AIS [50].

L-PAG-SPA is augmented by AIS lesioning and is completely inhibited by stimulation via the lesioning electrodes inserted in the AIS. D-PAG-SPA, however, is not influenced by this method of lesioning and stimulation. Augmentation of the L-PAG-SPA is only observed when the stimulating electrodes are located in the caudal L-PAG. When they are located in the rostral L-PAG, this augmentation is not observed. Therefore, the sites of the inhibitory action of the AIS on the pathway connected to the NAP are determined to be situated between the rostral and caudal L-PAG [41].

Chronic administration of large doses of morphine abolished both AA and MA (0.5 mg/kg). However, following AIS lesioning, analgesia was re-induced by stimulation of the AP [51, 52]. Teitelbaum et al. reported that EEG changes induced by repeat morphine injections become similar to the normal arousal pattern by lesioning the medial thalamus [83].

The inhibitory action of the AIS on NAA and the connections of the AP and NAP to the different afferent pathways were further confirmed by recording potentials from the D-PAG, L-PAG, L-CM, and I-PH evoked by stimulation of the AP and NAP [20]. Potentials were evoked specifically in the D-PAG by stimulation of the AP (tibial muscle), but not by that of the NAP (abdominal muscle). Potentials were nonspecifically evoked in the L-PAG by stimulation of the NAP as well as the AP. Evoked potentials in the L-PAG were depressed gradually by 1-Hz stimulation of the AP and NAP and were completely abolished 10 min after onset of stimulation. This depression in the L-PAG-evoked potentials disappeared after lesioning an area of the AIS, such as the L-CM, while potentials evoked in the D-PAG by AP stimulation did not change during stimulation of the NAP [20] (Fig. 13).

Potentials were evoked in areas of the AIS, such as the L-CM and I-PH, by stimulation of the AP and NAP. Therefore the AIS is activated by stimulation of either point. Potentials evoked in the L-PAG by stimulation of the AP and NAP were completely inhibited by AIS stimulation. This inhibition was observed when the recording electrodes were located in the rostral L-PAG, but not when located in the caudal L-PAG. Therefore, NAA is inhibited by the AIS between the rostral and caudal L-PAG (AP: 5.6 in Pregrino Cushman brain atlas). Inhibition of the L-PAG-evoked potential during stimulation of the I-PH was abolished by prior L-CM lesioning. Thus, the AIS originates from the AP as well as the NAP, ascends to the I-PH, passes through the L-CM, and reaches the L-PAG which is inhibited by the AIS [20, 41]. The specificity of the acupuncture point in producing AA is thus attributed to the fact that the AP is connected to a specific analgesia-producing pathway. The NAP is connected to another pathway that is inhibited by the AIS. The AIS in turn is nonspecifically activated by stimulation of the AP as well as by stimulation of the NAP. Hence, analgesia, normally induced only by stimulating the AP, was also achieved by stimulating the NAP only after lesioning the AIS.

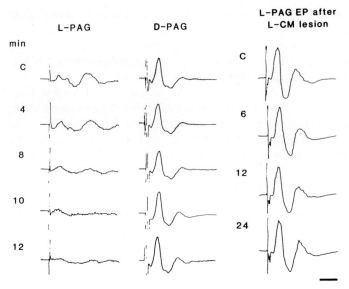

Fig. 13. Evoked potentials from a typical rat in L-PAG were gradually depressed and finally abolished by 1-Hz repetitive stimulation of the acupuncture point *(left);* those in the D-PAG were not influenced *(middle).* After lesioning the L-CM, inhibition of evoked potentials in the L-PAG disappeared *(right). Numbers* by each record indicate time in minutes after start of stimulation (20 ms [20]

In addition to the neuroanatomical differences in these two pathways, their pharmacological properties are also different. NAA is also induced after DPA (250 mg/kg) treatment and after treatment with the cholecystokinin antagonist, proglumide (20 µg/kg) [80]. Inhibition of both the NAP and AP stimulation induced analgesia after lesioning the AAP and during stimulation of the AIS is completely antagonized by DPA [17, 72]. Inhibition by stimulation of the AIS of both the L-PAG potentials evoked by 1-Hz repetitive stimulation of the AP and NAP and the L-PAG potentials evoked before starting repetitive stimulation is completely antagonized by DPA [20]. When DPA (84 µg) or proglumide (8 ng) are injected into the AIS directly, a similar form of analgesia is induced by stimulation of the NAP as that after AIS lesioning [80]. Both DPA and proglumide have no effect on the L-PAG. Therefore, DPA and proglumide directly inhibit the AIS. It is suggested that cholecystokinin (CCK) is the transmitter in the I-PH and L-CM of the AIS. The relationship between CCK and DPA has not yet been determined.

In this context DPA has two actions: one is the inhibition of either enkephalinase or aminopeptidase thus abolishing the individual variation in effectiveness, and the other is a direct inhibition on the AIS thus inducing NAA.

The ability of proglumide to potentiate morphine analgesia as reported by other investigators [87] can in part be explained by the existence of masked analgesia and the inhibitory action of proglumide on the AIS.

Pituitary and Adrenal Glands in Acupuncture and Nonacupuncture Stimulation Produced Analgesia

Removal of the pituitary or adrenal glands completely abolishes AA and NAA. However, augmentation of the AA, NAA, and SPA of the AAP appears 6 h after removal of these glands [58]. Abolition of the AA and the AAP-SPA takes 12 h, while that of NAA takes 16 h. The augmented analgesia is not blocked by either naloxone or dexamethasone but is blocked by lesioning an AAP area, such as the D-PAG, and by administering an AEP antagonist. Potentials evoked in the D-PAG by AP stimulation disappear concurrently with the abolition of AA after removal of the adrenal gland [58].

Analgesia was induced by morphine microinjection into the HARN, which was explored as the initital region of the descending pain inhibitory system in AA (unpublished observation). AA and SPA of the anterior hypothalamus (AH$_2$-SPA), which is thought to be the final region of the AAP, was blocked by intraventicular injection of antiserum to β-endorphin [81]. Therefore, it is probable that the HARN is activated by β-endorphin, although the source of the β-endorphin released by AH$_2$ stimulation is not yet known [70]. Analgesia induced by morphine microinjection into the HARN was not influenced by removal of the adrenal gland (unpublished observation).

Therefore, some neurohumoral factor from the pituitary gland may modulate the transmission in the AAP, although such a humoral factor has not yet been determined. Existence of a neurohumoral factor in producing AA was proved by a crossed circulation experiment evaluating the characteristic EEG changes in the deep brain of rabbits during acupuncture stimulation [76]. Since all SPAs of the AAP are naloxone reversible, opioid neuronal transmissions, such as enkephalinergic and endorphinergic transmissions, might be modulated by this kind of neurohumoral factor.

Relationship of Shock-Induced Analgesia to Acupuncture Analgesia

Analgesia is induced by electrical stress shock (1-s duration at 0.2 Hz) applied to the upper part of the lower extremities (SIA) [86]. This analgesia is abolished by naloxone, dexamethasone, hypophysectomy, and adrenectomy as reported by Lewis et al. [37]. Like NAA, SIA is abolished by lesioning the L-PAG; however, AIS lesioning has no effect on SIA. Tolerance in SIA persists for 5 days. During this SIA-suppressed state, response to AA and NAA is similar to the control, and ITh administered naloxone has no effect on SIA [86]. Therefore, AA and NAA are effected by a different analgesia-producing system than that of SIA (Fig. 12). It was reported that corticosterone restores the abolished SIA after adrenectomy [43]; however, corticosterone does not restore AA or NAA [58].

Mechanism of Muscle Pain Relief by Acupuncture

It has been clinically reported that needle insertion into the acupuncture point is effective in relieving pain in spastic muscles. This needling effect might be attributed to the improvement of the reduced circulation in the spastic muscle, since it was clinically reported that the lowered temperature in spastic muscle was returned to a normal temperature by acupuncture needle insertion [26]. The reduced circulation of spastic muscle might lead to the accumulation of pain-causing substances in the ischemic state. Under these conditions, ischemic pain is produced by muscular movement [67]. Improvement of the circulation should eliminate these pain substances.

This concept was proved by an experimental model of ischemic muscle pain. The isometric twitch height of the guinea pig gastrocnemius muscle in situ was gradually reduced to about half that of the control by tetanic stimulation (10 Hz) of the muscle for 60 min. We assume that this state of reduced twitch approximates that during ischemic pain production.

Pain Relief by Needle Insertion into the Spastic Muscle

Oblique needle insertion into the tetanized muscle immediately following tetanic stimulation facilitated recovery from the reduced twitch height, which was almost completely restored within about 2 h, while the control twitch without needling remained at a reduced height. Longitudinal needle insertion parallel to the muscle fibers was less effective in restoring the reduced twitch height [27, 34].

Recovery of twitch height may be attributed to improvement of the reduced circulation, since it can easily be supposed that the twitch height is depressed by the ischemic state. Perhaps the accumulated pain substances could thus be eliminated.

Cutting the sciatic nerve does not influence this needling effect (which facilitated the recovery of the reduced twitch height), but the needling effect is abolished by denervation [28, 63], IV administered atropine (0.5 mg), and capsaicin (50, 100, 200, and 400 μg/kg during 5 days' treatment) [28]. Therefore, the axon reflex and the cholinergic vasodilator nerve leading to the blood vessel in the muscle might be involved in the production of this needling effect.

Intra-arterial injection of saline (0.3–1.0 ml) and a vasodilator, such as isoproterenol (60 ng in 0.1 ml) or prostaglandin E_2 (10 ng in 0.1 ml), into the muscle produced a similar effect to that of needling into tetanized muscle. This shows that improvement of the reduced circulation is brought about by needle insertion into the muscle. Stimulation of the sciatic nerve under d-tubocurarine treatment also produced a similar effect to that of needling. This effect was abolished by intra-arterial atropine [34].

Since capsaicin abolishes the needling effect, the small primary afferent nerve is presumed to be involved [44]. Intra-arterial injection of a transmitter of a primary afferent nerve, such as substance P (10 nM) or calcitonin-gene-related peptide (CGRP; 10 nM) produces an effect similar to that of needling. The effect of CGRP is blocked by atropine and is not influenced by d-tubocurarine, but that of substance P is not blocked by atropine [34].

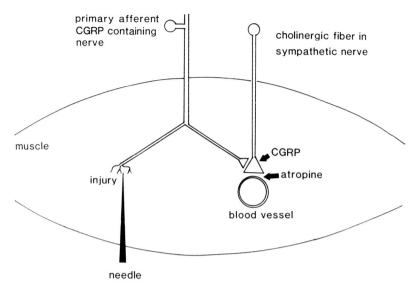

Fig. 14. The pain relief mechanism of needle insertion into the painful muscle. Needle insertion stimulates the nerve endings of the calcitonin-gene-related peptide *(CGRP)*-containing primary afferent nerve. Its axon collaterals innervate the nerve endings of the cholinergic nerve ending in the sympathetic nerve leading to the blood vessel and excite them. The release of acetylcholine is facilitated by the needle insertion, which produces dilation of the blood vessel in the spastic ischemic muscle [34]

Löfstirow et al. reported that the vasodilator activity of substance P is not influenced by atropine and that substance P might act on the blood vessel directly [40]. The intense vasodilator action of CGRP was reported by Brain et al. [8].

A schema to explain the effect of needle insertion on relieving muscle pain in thus proposed as shown in Fig. 14. Needle insertion stimulates the CGRP-containing, primary afferent nerve endings. Their axon collaterals innervate the nerve endings of the cholinergic vasodilator nerve in the sympathetic nerve. The release of acetylcholine from the cholinergic nerve to dilate the blood vessel is facilitated by needle insertion through these nerve ending connections. Therefore, the pain-stricken muscle itself is the acupuncture point for relieving muscle pain.

Pain Relief by Needle Insertion into the Acupuncture Point

Recovery of the reduced twitch of the gastrocnemius muscle after tetanic stimulation can be induced by another procedure, needle insertion into the ipsilateral L4/S1 perivertebral muscles [63] (Fig. 15). Insertion of the needle into the skin over the area has no effect on the twitch height. This needling effect is abolished by cutting the sciatic nerve, caudal lesioning by knife cut to the anterior hypothalamus, and IV injection of atropine 0.1 mg/kg. The rostral lesioning by knife cut to the anterior hypothalamus does not influence this effect. Focal electrical stimulation of the restricted region (0.7–1.0 mm lateral) in the anterior hypothalamus

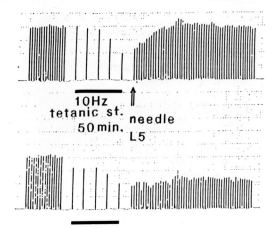

Fig. 15. Facilitation of recovery from reduced twitch after tetanic stimulation by needle insertion into the perivertebral muscle. Twitch heights of both sides of the gastrocnemius muscle of guinea pigs in situ were reduced after 50 min of 10-Hz tetanic stimulation. Needle insertion to the L5 perivertebral muscle facilitated the recovery of the ipsilateral reduced twitch, and produced almost complete recovered within 2 h, while that of the contralateral remained reduced [63]

(1–2.5 mm above the optic chiasma) produces an effect similar to that of needling into the contralateral perivertebral muscle [33].

Eliasson et al. reported that stimulation of the area close to the midline in the anterior hypothalamus (1–2 mm above the optic chiasma) of cats elicits bilateral vasodilation in the skeletal muscle of the hind leg due to activation of the sympathetic cholinergic nerve [14]. In personal experiments, the facilitation of recovery from reduced twitch height of the gastrocnemius muscle, which was presumed to be induced by recovery of the circulation, was unilateral. Eliasson et al., at a more intense level, stimulated with 2-ms, 1-4-V pulses (electrode resistance 1000 Ω) at a frequency of 70 per s [14]. I used milder stimulation with 600 μs duration at 80 Hz, gradually increasing during 600 ms to a maximum intensity of 200 μA with a repetition rate of 1 per s. Mild stimulation prevents current spread to the opposite side whereas intense midline stimulation might influence the neurons on both sides.

Potentials were evoked from the electrodes inserted into the anterior hypothalamus by stimulation through the needle inserted in the contralateral perivertebral muscle, which induced an acupuncture effect [33]. Therefore, this acupuncture needling effect was produced by a somato-autonomic reflex. The schema of this reflex is shown in Fig. 16. The effective sites of the needling into the perivertebral muscle for circulation of the gastrocnemius muscle were distributed widely from L4 to S1. Although all of the affected muscles responding to such stimulation of the L4/S1 perivertebral muscle were not checked, as far as the improvement of the circulation of the pain-stricken gastrocnemius muscle was concerned, the acupuncture effective sites were not restricted to one point but were spread over a wide region.

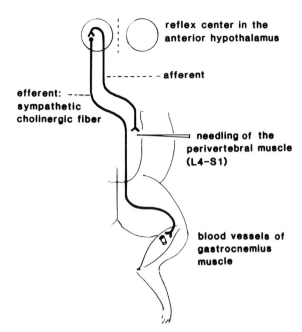

Fig. 16. Gastrocneumius muscle pain relief mechanism of needle insertion into the perivertebral muscle. Needle insertion into the perivertebral muscle (L4/S1) stimulates the somatic nerve endings in the muscle. Afferent impulses initiating from these nerve endings ascend to the controlateral anterior hypothalamus. Efferent impulses in the cholinergic vasodilator nerve originate from the reflex center in the anterior hypothalamus (intervening synapses not shown) descend to the contralateral gastrocnemius muscle, and dilate the blood vessel in the spastic ischemic muscle. This needling effect is due to the somato-autonomic reflex. The reflex center is located in the anterior hypothalamus [33]

Summary

The mechanism of AA induced by low-frequency stimulation of the muscle corresponding to the acupuncture point is described, based on the results of animal experiments.

Individual variations in effectiveness of AA are mostly evident in the sensitive opioid transmission site in the spinal cord of the AAP from the AP to the hypophysis, although individual variation in effectiveness was observed in all stimulation-produced analgesias throughout the AAP.

Acupuncture points and nonacupuncture points are distinguished by the differing central pathways. The pathway connected to the nonacupuncture point is inhibited by the AIS, which is activated by stimulation of the AP as well as the NAP. Both D-phenylalanine and proglumide directly inhibit the AIS.

The descending pain inhibitory system is activated in AA as the AEP. This system is common in producing AA, NAP-SPA after lesioning of the AIS, and in electrical stress SIA.

Pain originating in the spastic gastrocnemius muscle is relieved by improvement of the reduced circulation after needle insertion into the gastrocnemius or the ipsilateral L4/S1 perivertebral muscle. The former effect is induced by an axon reflex in the nerve terminals of the CGRP-containing primary afferent nerve, and the latter effect is induced by a somato-autonomic reflex, the center of which lies in the anterior hypothalamus.

References

1. Abbott FV, Melzack R (1978) Analgesia produced by stimulation of limbic structures and its relation to epileptiform after-discharges. Exp Neurol 62: 730-734
2. Akaike A, Shibata T, Satoh M, Takagi H (1978) Analgesia induced by microinjection of morphine into, and electrical stimulation of the nucleus reticularis paragigantocellularis of rat medulla oblongata. Neuropharmacology 17: 775-778
3. Andersson SA, Ericson T, Holmgren E, Lindqvist G (1973 Electro-acupuncture effect on pain threshold measured with electrical stimulation of teeth. Brain Res 63: 393-396
4. Andersson SA, Holmgren E (1975) On acupuncture analgesia and mechanism of pain. Am J Chin Med 3: 331-334
5. Atweh SF, Kuhar MJ (1977) Autoradiographic localization of opiate receptors in rat brain: II. The brainstem. Brain Res 129: 1-12
6. Balagura S, Ralph T (1973) The analgesic effect of electrical stimulation of the diencephalon and mesencephalon. Brain Res 60: 369-379
7. Bloom F, Battenberg E, Rossier J, Ling N, Guillemin R (1978) Neurons containing β-endorphin in rat brain exist separately from those containing enkephalin: immunocytochemical studies. Proc Natl Acad Sci (USA) 75: 1591-1595
8. Brain SD, Williams TJ, Tippins JR, Morris HR, MacIntyre I (1985) Calcitonin gene-related peptide is a potent vasodilator. Nature 313: 54-56
9. Breglio V, Anderson DC, Merrill HK (1970) Alteration in footshock threshold by low-level septal brain stimulation. Physiol Behav 5: 715-719
10. Cheng R, Pomeranz B, Yu G (1979) Dexamethasone partially reduces and saline-treatment abolished alectroacupuncture analgesia: these findings implicate pituitary endorphins. Life Sci 24: 1481-1486
11. Cheng R, Pomeranz B (1979) Electroacupuncture analgesia could be mediated by at least two pain-relieving mechanisms: endorphin and non-endorphin systems. Life Sci 25: 1957-1962
12. Chiang CY, Chang CT (1973) Peripheral afferent pathway for acupuncture analgesia. Sci Sin 16: 210-217
13. Cox VC, Valenstein ES (1965) Attenuation of aversive properties of peripheral shock by hypothalamic stimulation. Science 149: 323-325
14. Eliasson S, Folkow B, Lindgren P, Uvnas B (1951) Activation of sympathetic vasodilator nerves to the skeletal muscle in the cat by hypothalamic stimulation. Acta Physiol Scand 23: 333-351
15. Fu TC, Halenda SP, Dewey WL (1980) The effect of hypophysectomy on acupuncture analgesia in the mouse. Brain Res 202: 33-39
16. Fujishita Y, Hisamitsu M, Takeshige C (1981) Difference between non-acupuncture point stimulation-produced and acupuncture analgesia after D-phenylalanine treatment. J Showa Med Assoc, 41, 657-662
17. Fujishita Y, Murai M, Takeshige C (1986) Inhibition of acupuncture and morphine analgesia caused by posterior hypothalamic stimulation and antagonistic action of D-phenylalanine in inhibition. J Showa Med Assoc 45: 799-805
18. Gol A (1967) Relief of pain by electrical stimulation of the septal area. J Neurol Sci 5: 115-120
19. Hisamitsu T (1979) Role of limbic system in acupuncture anesthesia: I. Analysis of evoked potential in limbic system induced by acupuncture stimulation. J Showa Med Assoc 38: 551-557
20. Hishida F, Luo CP, Okubo K, Takeshige C (1986) Differentiation of acupuncture point and non-acupuncture point explored by evoked potential of the central nervous system and its correlation with analgesia inhibitory system. J Showa Med Assoc 46: 35-43
21. Hishida F, Okamoto T, Takeshige C (1987) Individual variations in effectiveness of acupunc-

ture analgesia evaluated by evoked potential in the dorsal periaqueductal central gray and effect of D-phenylalanine. J Showa Med Assoc 47: 153–158

22. Hishida F, Tanaka M, Mera T, Jauwhie, J, Takeshige C (1986) Effects of D-phenylalanine on individual variation of analgesia and on analgesia inhibitory system in their separated experimental procedures. J Showa Med Assoc 46: 45–51

23. Ito H (1981) Involvement of dopaminergic system in acupuncture analgesia. J Showa Med Assoc 41: 165–170

24. Jauwhie J, Sato T, Hisamitsu T, Takeshige C (1986) Acupuncture afferent and efferent pathways in the reticulogigantocellular nucleus and reticuloparagigantocellular nucleus. J Showa Med Assoc 46: 65–73

25. Kawakita K (1981) Role of the polymodal receptors in acupuncture analgesia of the rat. Comp Med East-West 6 (4): 312–321

26. Kinoshita H (1981) Experimental research of acupuncture effect on local pain: I. Mechanism of acupuncture-moxibustion's effect on local pain estimated from skin and muscle temperatures and volume pulse wave. J Showa Med Assoc 41: 147–156

27. Kinoshita H (1981) Experimental research of acupuncture effect on local pain: II. Effect of stationary insertion on the contraction recovery process following tetanus. J Showa Med Assoc 41: 393–403

28. Kinoshita H (1981) Experimental research of acupuncture effect on local pain: III. Effect of acupuncture in recovery from reduced muscle contraction of tetanized muscle and its correlation with conditions of acupuncture needling. J Showa Med Assoc 41: 405–409

29. Kobayashi RM, Palkovits M, Miller RJ, Chang KJ, Cuatrecasas P (1978) Brain enkephalin distribution is unaltered by hypophysectomy. Life Sci 22: 527–530

30. Kobori M, Mera H, Takeshige C (1981) Central acupuncture afferent pathways. J Showa Med Assoc 41: 619–628

31. Kobori M, Mera H, Takeshige C (1982) Nature of acupuncture point and non-point stimulation produced analgesia after lesion of analgesia inhibitory system. J Showa Med Assoc 42: 589–598

32. Kuhar MJ, Pert CB, Snyder SH (1973) Regional distribution of opiate receptor binding in monkey and human brain. Nature 245: 447–450

33. Kusumoto S, Sato M, Takeshige C (1985) The experimental research on acupuncture effect on local muscle pain: V. The reflex center of acupuncture needling effect of perivertebral muscle on the recovery from reduced twitch in the gastrocnemius muscle after tetanic stimulation. J Showa Med Assoc 45: 279–285

34. Kuwazawa J, Sato M, Takeshige C (1987) Experimental research of acupuncture effect on local muscle pain: VI. Effect of vasodilators and neuropeptide on recovery from the reduced twitch after tetanic stimulation. J Showa Med Assoc 47: 15–22

35. Le Bars D, Dickenson AH, Besson JM (1979) Diffuse noxious inhibitory controls (DNIC): I. Effects on dorsal horn convergent neurons in the rat. Pain 6: 283–304

36. Le Bars D, Dickenson AH, Besson JM (1979) Diffuse noxious inhibitory controls (DNIC): II. Lack of effect on non-convergent neurons, supraspinal involvement and theoretical implications. Pain 6: 305–327

37. Lewis JW (1986) Multiple neurochemical and hormonal mechanisms of stress-induced analgesia. Ann NY Acad Sci 457: 194–204

38. Lewis JW, Cannon JT, Liebeskind JC (1980) Opioid and non-opioid mechanisms of stress analgesia. Science 208: 623–625

39. Lo FS, Yuan CS, Yaung SL, Tuanmu CH, Chang HT (1979) Inhibition of nociceptive discharges of parafascicular neurons by direct electrical stimulation of nucleus centrum medianum. Sci Sin 21 (4): 533–535

40. Löfstrom B, Pernow B, Wahren J (1965) Vasodilating action of substance P in the human forearm. Acta Physiol Scand 63: 311–324

41. Luo CP, Hishida F, Kusumoto S, Takeshige C (1983) Inhibited region by analgesia inhibitory system in acupuncture non-point stimulation-produced analgesia. J Showa Med Assoc 43: 609–613

42. Luo CP, Sato M, Shimizu S, Takeshige C (1979) Role of limbic system in acupuncture analgesia: II. Role of septal nucleus and cingulate bundle in acupuncture and morphine analgesia. J Showa Med Assoc 39: 559–568

43. MacLennan AJ, Crugan RC, Hyson RL, Maier SF (1982) Corticosterone: a critical factor in opioid form of stress-induced analgesia. Science 215: 1530-1532
44. Matsuyama T, Wanaka A, Yoneda S, Kimura K, Kamada T, Girgis S, Macintyre I, Emson PC, Tohyama M (1986) Two distinct calcitonin gene-related peptide-containing peripheral nervous systems: distribution and quantitative differences between the iris and cerebral artery with special reference to substancce P. Brain Res 373: 205-212
45. Mayer DJ, Liebeskind JC (1974) Pain reduction by focal electrical stimulation of the brain: an anatomical and behavioral analysis. Brain Res 68: 73-93
46. Mayer DJ, Price DD, Rafii A (1977) Antagonism of acupuncture analgesia in man by narcotic antagonist naloxone. Brain Res 121: 369-372
47. Mayer DJ, Wolfle TL, Akil H, Carder B, Liebeskind JC (1971) Analgesia from electrical stimulation in the brainstem of the rat. Science 174: 1351-1354
48. Menetrey D, Giesler Jr GJ, Besson JM (1977) An analysis of response properties of spinal cord dorsal horn neurons to non-noxious and noxious stimuli in the spinal rat. Exp Brain Res 27: 15-33
49. Mera T (1987) The paragigantocellular nucleus as the descending pain inhibitory system in acupuncture analgesia. J Showa Med Assoc 47: 89-97
50. Mera H, Kobori M, Takeshige C (1981) Acupuncture and morphine analgesia inhibitory system in the lateral centromedian nucleus of the thalamus. J Showa Med Assoc 41: 629-640
51. Mera H, Kobori M, Takeshige C (1981) Relationship between acupuncture, morphine tolerance and analgesia inhibitory system. J Showa Med Assoc 41: 641-645
52. Mera H, Kobori M, Takeshige C (1981) Differentiation between acupuncture analgesia producing central system and analgesia producing system inhibited by analgesia inhibitory system by different production of morphine tolerance. J Showa Med Assoc 42: 599-604
53. Mizuno T, Takahashi G (1982) Abolishment of acupuncture analgesia measured by vocalization after hypophysectomy. J Showa Med Assoc 42: 427-431
54. Mizuno T (1982) The nature of acupuncture point investigated by evoked potential from the dorsal periaqueductal central gray in acupuncture afferent pathway. J Showa Med Assoc 42: 417-425
55. Ogawa N, Panerai AE, Lee S, Forsbach G, Havlicek V, Friesen HG (1979) β-endorphin concentration in the brain of intact and hypophysectomized rats. Life Sci 25: 317-326
56. Oka K (1979) Abolishment of acupuncture analgesia by partial lesion of periaqueductal central gray. J Showa Med Assoc 39: 397-407
57. Oka K, Takeshige C (1979) Effect of acupuncture or periaqueductal central gray stimulation on noxious responses in brainstem reticular formation neurons. J Showa Med Assoc 39: 569-580
58. Okubo K (1987) Effect of the pituitary or adrenal gland ablation on analgesia caused by the acupuncture point stimulation or non-acupuncture point stimulation after lesion of the analgesia inhibitory system. J Showa Med Assoc 47: 99-106
59. Pert CB, Snyder SH (1973) Opiate receptor: demonstration in nervous tissue. Science 179: 1011-1014
60. Poitras D, Parent A (1978) Atlas of the distribution of monoamine-containing nerve cell bodies in the brain stem of the cat. J Comp Neurol 179: 699-718
61. Pomeranz B, Chiu D (1976) Naloxone blockade of acupuncture analgesia: endorphin implicated. Life Sci 19: 1757-1762
62. Rhodes DL, Liebeskind JC (1978) Analgesia from rostral brain stem stimulation in the rat. Brain Res 143: 521-532
63. Sato M, Takeshige C (1982) Experimental research on acupuncture effect on local pain: IV. Effect of acupuncture application on perivertebral muscle in the recovery process from reduced twitch of gastrocnemius muscle after tetanic stimulation. J Showa Med Assoc 42: 441-447
64. Sato T, Takeshige C (1981) Morphine analgesia caused by activation of spinal acupuncture afferent pathway in the anterolateral tract: experimental study of extradural analgesia. J Showa Med Assoc 41: 663-673
65. Sato T, Usami S, Takeshige C (1983) Role of the arcuate nucleus of the hypothalamus as the descending pain inhibitory system in acupuncture point and non-point stimulation produced analgesia. J Showa Med Assoc 43: 619-627

66. Sato T, Mera T, Abe M, Takeshige C (1986) The ventromedian nucleus of the hypothalamus as the descending pain inhibitory system. J Showa Med Assoc 46: 59–64
67. Sicuteri F, Franchi G, Michelacci S (1974) Biochemical mechanism of ischemic pain. Adv Neurol 4: 39–44
68. Sjolund BH, Eriksson MBE (1979) The influence of naloxone on analgesia produced by peripheral conditioning stimulation. Brain Res 173: 295–301
69. Sjolund BH, Eriksson BE (1979) Endorphins and analgesia produced peripheral conditioning stimulation. Adv Pain Res Ther 3: 587–592
70. Sjolund B, Terenius L, Eriksson M (1977) Increased cerebrospinal fluid levels of endorphins after electroacupuncture. Acta Physiol Scand 160: 382–384
71. Snyder SH (1975) Opiate receptor in normal and drug altered brain function. Nature 257: 185–189
72. Takahashi G, Mera H, Kobori M (1983) Inhibitory action on analgesic inhibitory system and augmenting action on naloxone reversible analgesia of D-phenylalanine. J Showa Med Assoc 43: 603–608
73. Takahashi G, Usami S, Kusumoto S (1983) Abolishment of analgesia in acupuncture anesthesia measured by writing test after hypophysectomy. J Showa Med Assoc 43: 615–618
74. Takeshige C (1987) Inhibition associated with acupuncture analgesia. Neurol Neurobiol 28: 255–262
75. Takeshige C (1985) Differentiation between acupuncture and non-acupuncture points by association with analgesia inhibitory system. Acupunct Elektrother Res 10: 195–203
76. Takeshige C, Luo CP, Kamada Y (1976) Modulation of EEG and unit discharges of deep structures of brain during acupuncture stimulation and hypnosis of rabbits. Adv Pain Res Therap 1: 781–785
77. Takeshige C, Mera H, Kobori M, Sato T, Luo CP (1981) Afferent and efferent pathways in acupuncture analgesia and their correlation with morphine analgesia. Adv. Endogenous and Exogenous Opioids, Proceeding of the International Narcotic Research Conference, Kyoto, Japan. July 26–30, 1981 Kodansha Ltd, Tokyo, pp 291–293
78. Takeshige C, Murai M, Tanaka M, Hachisu M (1983) Parallel individual variations in effectiveness of acupuncture, morphine analgesia, and dorsal PAG-SPA and their abolition by D-phenylalanine. Adv Pain Res, Ther 5: 563–569
79. Takeshige C, Sato T, Komugi H (1980) Role of periaqueductal central gray in acupuncture analgesia. Acupunct Electrother Res 5: 323–337
80. Tanaka M, Igarashi O, Hisamitsu T, Takeshige C (1988) Effect of D-phenylalanine and proglumide on analgesia inhibitory system. J Showa Med Assoc (In press)
81. Tanaka M, Murai M, Okubo K, Jauwhie J, Takeshige C (1985) Abolition of analgesia caused by low frequency acupuncture stimulation after intraventricular application of anti-serum of β-endorphin. J Showa Med Assoc 46: 53–58
82. Tanaka M, Sato T, Okamoto T, Takeshige C (1987) Morphine analgesia mediated by activation of the acupuncture afferent pathway as evaluation of the dose response relationship. J Showa Med Assoc 47: 159–166
83. Teitelbaum H, Catravas GN, McFarland WL (1974) Reversal of morphine tolerance after medial thalamis lesions in the rat. Science 185: 449–451
84. Toda K, Ichioka M (1978) Electroacupuncture: relations between forelimb afferent impulses and suppression of jaw-opening reflex elicited by tooth pulp stimulation. Jpn J Physiol 28: 485–497
85. Tsuruoka M (1987) Suppression of the tail flick reflex by A afferent nerve impulses. J Showa Med Assoc 43: 43–55
86. Usami S, Takeshige C (1983) The difference in analgesia producing central pathway of stress induced analgesia and that of acupuncture point and non-pont stimulation-produced analgesia. J Showa Med Assoc 43: 629–638
87. Watkins LR, Kinscheck IB, Mayer DJ (1985) Potentiation of morphine analgesia by the cholecystokinin antagonist proglumide. Brain Res 327: 169–180
88. Watkins LR, Mayer DJ (1982) Organization of endogenous opiate and nonopiate pain control systems. Science 216: 1185–1192
89. Watkins LR, Cobelli DA, Newsome HH, Mayer DJ (1982) Footshock induced analgesia is dependent neither on pituitary nor sympathetic activation. Brain Res 245: 81–96

90. Willcockson WS, Kim J, Shin HK, Chung JM, Willis WD (1986) Actions of opioids on primate spinothalamic tract neurons. J Neurosci 6: 2509–2520
91. Woolf CJ, Barrett GD, Mitchell D, Myers RA (1977) Naloxone-reversible peripheral electroanalgesia in intact and spinal rats. Eur J Pharmacol 45: 311–314
92. Woolf CJ, Mitchell D, Barrett GD (1980) Antiociceptive effect of peripheral segmental electrical stimulation in the rat. Pain 8: 237–252
93. Yaksh TL (1978) Analgesic action of intrathecal opiates in cat and primate. Brain Res 153: 205–210
94. Yaksh TL, Rudy TA (1976) Analgesia mediated by a direct spinal action of narcotics. Science 192: 1357–1358
95. Yaksh TL, Rudy RA (1977) Studies on the direct spinal action of narcotics in the production of analgesia in the rat. J Pharmacol Exp Ther 202: 411–428
96. Yaksh TL, Yeung JC, Rudy TA (1976) Systemic examination in the rat of brain stem sites sensitive to the direct application of morphine: observation of differential effects within the periaqueductal gray. Brain Res 114: 83–103
97. Yeung JC, Yaksh TL, Rudy TA (1975) Effects of brain lesions on the antinociceptive properties of morphine in rats. Clin Exp Pharmacol Physiol 2: 261–268

Neurophysiological Mechanisms Involved in the Pain-Relieving Effects of Counterirritation and Related Techniques Including Acupuncture

D. Le Bars[1], J. C. Willer[2], T. de Broucker[2], and L. Villanueva[1]

[1] INSERM U-161, 2, rue d'Alésia, 75014 Paris, France
[2] Dept. Physiol., Lab. Neurophysiol., Faculté Médecine Pitié-Salpêtrière, 91, Bd. de l'Hôpital, 75013 Paris, France

Counterirritation phenomena, i.e., the paradoxical, pain-relieving effects of painful stimulation of heterotopic areas of the body have been known for centuries, and various non-Western (e.g., Chinese) medical procedures still include counterirritation as a pain-relieving technique. In fact, most "popular" methods of practising medicine include the therapeutic use of counterirritation [95], and it has been repeatedly rediscovered by scientists!

In the present review, we will first briefly consider clinical and experimental observations in man and behavioral experiments in animals which support the notion that "pain inhibits pain." Thereafter, a neural substrate for this phenomenon will be proposed on the basis of electrophysiological experiments in both man and animals. In the final section evidence for the involvement of such mechanisms in pain management by somatic stimulation will be discussed.

Clinical Observations

Most counterirritant procedures have involved the production of a more or less bearable level of pain as a treatment for preexistent pain. In 1956, Wand-Tetley reviewed a series of old counterirritation methods used for the treatment of rheumatic diseases [137]. Most of them were undoubtedly painful: for instance, "cupping" when associated with scarification of the skin, cautery, moxibustion, or blisters. Another example was the use of discharge from the electric eel for the relief of pain. As reviewed by Kane and Taub [68], the Greeks and probably the Egyptians knew about these effects, which are referred to in numerous manuscripts.

Such clinical practices progressively disappeared in modern occidental medicine when analgesic and anti-inflammatory drugs became available. It should be stressed, however, that country people still use procedures such as twitch in horses and barnacles in cattle for surgical purposes (e.g., docking horse's tails, castrating calves) in the absence of any medication. The use of moxibustion in Chinese popular veterinary medicine is illustrated in Fig. 1.

The use of electrical stimulation was introduced in the 19th century as a pain-relieving method and, despite being a subject of controversy, it has commonly been used in Western medicine [68]. In the light of present neurophysiological knowledge, it appears that several mechanisms might have been brought into play by such techniques, depending on the nature of the current used and/or the part of the body to which it was applied. In some cases, segmental inhibitory mecha-

风湿症，是南方地区耕牛冬春多发的一种疾病。一般突然发病，肌肉疼痛，卧地，走路都较困难，手压腰部觉得板硬；也有关节突然肿胀、发热、疼痛的。按照发病部位不同，有腰风湿、四肢风湿和全身风湿等几种。

用针灸治疗风湿症，有明显疗效。民间还常用酒灸法来治疗，即用黄泥土或面糊等，在牛的百会穴处捏成一环状小圈，环中倾入烧酒，以火点燃，待酒烧尽，火即自熄。施术后，同时结合加强饲养与护理，注意栏舍保暖，多垫褥草，并给以含有丰富营养的饲料，如蛋壳粉、糠麸、酒糟、油饼等食用，则疗效更佳。

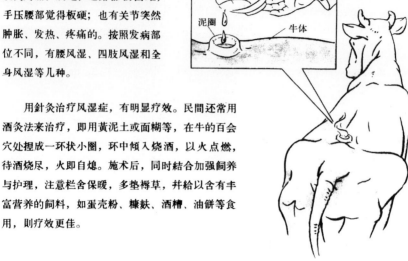

Fig. 1. Example of the technique of moxibustion as used in Chinese traditional veterinary practice to produce hypoalgesia (from a veterinary acupuncture plate sold in Peking in 1971). Translation: "In the south of China, draught cattle often exhibit rheumatic diseases in winter and spring. The symptoms appear suddenly with myalgia associated with lumbar stiffness and laborious walk. Lumbar, limb, or generalized rheumatisms are observed. Acupuncture is strongly effective against rheumatic syndromes. Popular treatment often uses moxibustion with alcohol: first one has to make a kind of ring using clay set on the lumbar 'Bai-Hui' point of the diseased cow; then alcohol is poured into it which must be consumed until extinction . . .". Note the implicit relevance in this text of acupuncture to the counter-irritation effects of an intense burn

nisms induced by low-intensity currents were most probably the underlying mechanisms. In others, the practices clearly involved counter-irritation phenomena [42, 115, 126].

More recently, painful electrical stimulation of the skin was reintroduced in the treatment of chronic pain [67, 94] and described as "hypoalgesia by hyperstimulation." Interestingly, the hypoalgesia induced by some forms of acupuncture or electroacupuncture has been postulated as being related to counter-irritation phenomena [47, 48, 86, 97, 137]. Based on wide clinical experience, the conclusion reached by Mann [91] was that acupuncture stimulation must be as strong as the patient can tolerate for a reliable pain-relieving effect to occur.

Finally, intense cold ("ice massage") applied to the hand has been reported to relieve dental pain [98], and related methods have been used for the treatment of muscular [56, 101] and low-back pain [99].

Further clinical evidence for the existence of a diffuse inhibitory system triggered by pain of peripheral origin is the observation that organic pain raises pain thresholds in other areas of the body [64, 89, 102].

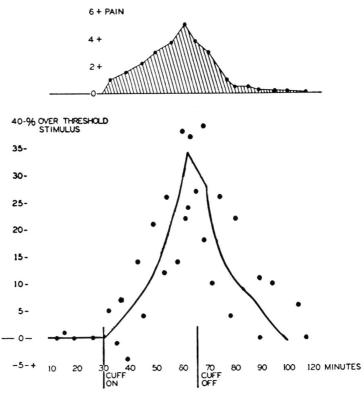

Fig. 2. The effect of arresting the blood flow to the left arm upon the pain threshold on the fore-head in man [61]. The *upper shaded area* represents the subjective estimates of the pain caused by ischemia in the arm (induced by a sphygmomanometer cuff wound above the elbow and inflated to a pressure of 200 mmHg). The pain threshold was estimated by applying thermal radiation to the forehead *(lower curve)*. Note that the pain sensation arising from the arm parallels the increase in the pain threshold from the forehead

Psychophysical Approaches in Man

To our knowledge, the first experimental investigation of counterirritation phe-nomena was made by Duncker [43]. Reffering to the practices we have mentioned above, he noted that "in the olden days where modern anaesthetics were not yet discovered, it was one of the functions of the dentist's assistant to pinch the pa-tient at the critical moment," and he undertook "experiments on the mutual influ-ence of pains" induced mechanically on right and left forearms. He concluded that in about 40 cases and without exception, a pain A ("active") induced a decrease of a distant and simultaneous pain P ("passive") if A was stronger than P and, if so, in proportion to A's relative intensity; interestingly, the pressure sensa-tion elicited by mild stimuli was not affected. Further experiments allowed him to conclude: "I never encountered any chance evidence that quality of A or distance between A and P were playing a part. Pain in a toe caused by contact with a hot-water bottle would readily yield under the influence of pain inflicted by pinching the lobe of an ear."

Hardy et al. [61] also reached similar conclusions. One of their experiments is illustrated in Fig. 2. The pain threshold was measured using radiant heat application to the forehead; a sphygmomanometer cuff placed around the left arm was then inflated to a pressure of 200 mmHg, which resulted in a progressive pain sensation associated with a disappearance of other sensations emanating from this arm. The threshold for pain elicited by means of thermal radiation of the forehead increased in a strikingly parallel fashion to the pain sensation elicited from the arm. Further investigations by the same group [9] using two radiant heat dolorimeters applied to various body areas confirmed these results and allowed them to state that both the pain and the reflex threshold were affected by what they called "extinction of pain."

Gammon and Starr [49], using several types of counter-irritants (cold, heat, mechanical, electrical), described a similar phenomenon, the most effective method being the application of painful cold ($4° - 10 °C$). They mainly investigated the effects of counter-irritants applied over the painful area (i.e., near the body surface where the conditioned painful stimulus was applied) but noticed that counter-irritation applied elsewhere was 'by no means ineffectual.' Similarly, Parsons and Goetzl [107] observed a rise in the threshold to dental pain during the application of a spray of ethyl chloride (nociceptive cold) to the anterior surface of the subject's tibiae. More recently, Pertovaara et al. [108] confirmed that pain resulting from ischemia of the arm associated with muscular exercise strongly increased the dental pain threshold and Talbot et al. [122] reported a reduced perception of painful heat stimuli on the face during and after the time the subjects submerged a hand in painfully cold water ($5°$). Our psychophysical observations, together with neurophysiological data, will be presented below.

Behavioral Approaches in Animals

The exprimental study of counterirritation phenomena in animals is not easy for several reasons. Apart from the general difficulties of studying pain in animals, there are problems related to the necessary application of two noxious stimuli – one "active" and affecting the response to the latter "passive" stimulus. Results may be influenced by the mutual effects of these stimuli [81], while the "active" stimulus might induce stress reactions other than those specifically related to nociception.

However, experimental data suggest that counter-irritation phenomena can be observed in animals. For instance, in the cat, stimulation of tooth pulp at an obviously noxious intensity can increase by up to 700% the threshold for escape behavior induced by footshock [3]. In rodents, sustained pinch applied to the paw or tail [30], noxious cold applied to the entire body [11], and various electrical shocks applied to the feet or tail [15, 16, 25, 63, 66, 87, 88, 125, 138, 139] can induce potent hypoalgesic effects. Visceral nociceptive stimuli can also induce hypoalgesia in behavioral testing [20, 24, 63, 71, 72]. In this respect, we have reported that a noxious peritoneovisceral stimulus [IP injection of phenylbenzoquinone (PBQ) or

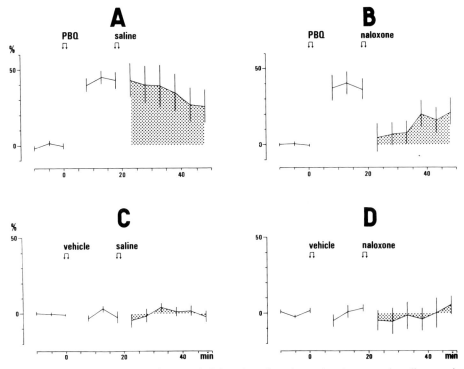

Fig. 3 A–D. Hypoalgesia elicited by IP administration of an algogenic substance, phenylbenzoquinone *(PBQ)* and its reversal by naloxone [71]. *Ordinate* shows percentage increase of the threshold for vocalization induced by electrical stimulation of the tail. **A** Control sequence for PBQ followed after 15 min by saline IV. **B** Reversal of PBQ effect by naloxone 200 µg/kg. **C** Evolution in vocalization threshold following PBQ vehicle and IV saline. **D** Effect of naloxone 200 µg/kg in the absence of a noxious conditioning stimulus. Note that while naloxone produced a very sharp threshold decrease in PBQ-treated animals, it had no significant effect in the unconditioned rat

acetic acid] produces a significant increase in the threshold for vocalization elicited by transcutaneous electrical stimulation of the tail. Conversely, the response (writhing) to the visceroperitoneal nociceptive stimulus is reduced in experimental arthritic rats during the most severe phase of the disease [19].

The time course for the PBQ effect on the vocalization threshold of normal rats is illustrated in Fig. 3A. As can be seen in Fig. 3B, naloxone 0.2 mg/kg IV antagonized this increase. This action was limited in time: 30 min after the injection of naloxone, the vocalization threshold returned to values comparable to those for PBQ-treated controls which received saline IV (Fig. 3C). Rats which received solvent alone as the conditioning injection were affected very little by this IV dose of naloxone (Fig. 3D).

These results show that a dull pain of peritoneovisceral origin can block the behavioral response to a focal peripheral stimulus and suggest the involvement of endogenous opioids in producing this effect. Interestingly twitch has been shown to increase, in a naloxone-reversible manner, the nociceptive threshold measured on the back of horses [74].

The participation of serotonergic mechanisms in counter-irritation phenomena has been investigated in the rat using the model described above. It was found that pretreatment with 5--hydroxytryptophan strongly potentiated, in a dose-dependent fashion, the PBQ-induced rise in threshold. The specificity of this effect was confirmed by its suppression by the serotonin receptor blocker, cinanserin [72].

Electrophysiological Approach in Man

In a recent study [146], we attempted to investigate counter-irritation phenomena in man using a combined psychophysical and neurophysiological approach. Knowing that the spinal cord is one of the main targets of most analgesic procedures [82], we postulated that counter-irritation phenomena may also act at this level.

A Spinal Target

To investigate this proposal, the sural nerve was stimulated in healthy volunteers and both the spinal RIII reflex and the simultaneously evoked sensation were recorded to study the effects of various conditioning nociceptive stimuli applied to the contralateral arm or nose of human subjects. This experimental protocol was chosen because the threshold of the RIII reflex had previously been found to be close to the threshold of pain [141].

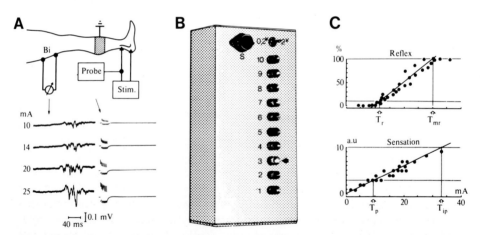

Fig. 4. A *Upper part,* experimental design for stimulating the sural nerve *(Stim.),* measuring the stimulus intensity *(Probe),* and recording the reflex activity from the biceps femoris muscle *(Bi). Lower part,* example of recruitment of the nociceptive reflex (RIII) activity *(left)* as a function of stimulus intensity *(right).* **B** Device used by the subjects for estimation of sensations elicited by the sural nerve stimuli. The 10-level visual scale consists of 10 potentiometers *(S output).* The pain threshold is defined as level 3 *(arrow)* and intolerable pain as level 10. **C** Examples of the intensity-response curves in the case of the reflex *(upper)* and sensation *(lower).* $T_r,$ reflex threshold; $T_{mr},$ threshold for obtaining a maximum reflex response; $T_p,$ pain threshold; $T_{ip},$ threshold for intolerable pain; *a.u.,* arbitrary units

The right sural nerve was stimulated at a rate of 0.25 Hz and the electromyographic reflex responses were recorded from the ipsilateral biceps femoris muscle (Fig. 4A). The subjective quality (tactile or painful) and intensity of the sensation elicited by the sural nerve stimulus were estimated by the subjects on the 10-level visual scale consisting of 10 switches (Fig. 4B) with the pain threshold being defined as level 3 and intolerable pain as level 10.

The intensity of stimulation was delivered randomly while both the digitized nociceptive reflex and sensation were plotted against stimulus intensity via a computer program. As shown in Fig. 4C, both the reflex activity and the subjective rating score increased linearly as a function of stimulus intensity within a limited range; this allowed the measurement of both pain and nociceptive reflex thresholds.

The experimental procedure consisted of sequences during which both the spinal nociceptive reflex (RIII) and the related subjective sensation elicited by stimulation of the right sural nerve were measured before and during the application of heterotopic conditioning somatic stimuli, e. g., immersion of the contralateral hand in a waterbath. As shown in Fig. 5, the responses were modified in direct relationship to the temperature of the waterbath. At 42 °C, neither the reflex nor the sensation curves were different from the controls. At 44 °C there was a slight shift to the right for the reflex response curve while the sensation curve remained unchanged. The shift of the reflex curve is mainly due to a change in the slope, the threshold being unchanged. By contrast, with 45°, 46° and 47 °C both the reflex and the sensation curves were shifted to the right, with a maximal effect for the highest temperature.

The intensity-reflex and intensity-sensation curves were also substantially shifted to the right by immersion of the contralateral hand in a 6 °C waterbath, by muscle pain induced by forearm muscular exercise during ischemia and by strong pressure applied to the nasal septum (Fig. 6).

In summary, these results demonstrate that experimentally induced pain can be profoundly modified by nociceptive stimuli applied to heterotopic body areas. In addition, these nociceptive conditioning stimuli were found to depress the simultaneously recorded nociceptive spinal reflex (RIII). With regard to the sensation or the reflex, both threshold and suprathreshold responses were affected; for thermal stimulation, this was directly related to the temperature applied within the nociceptive range.

It is worth pointing out the contrast between (a) the phasic nature of the conditioned (test) stimulus (20-ms electrical train) and the long duration (2–3 min) of the nociceptice conditioning stimuli; (b) the relatively restricted central input (part of S1) of the sural nerve compared with the wide distribution of the central inputs evoked by the various conditioning stimuli; and (c) the larger central somatotopic representation of the hand and the nose compared with that of the foot. There was therefore a clear imbalance between the afferent volleys triggered by the conditioning and the conditioned stimuli. Previous studies [143] have shown that the stimulation parameters used in the present work for eliciting a RIII reflex activate predominantly the myelinated fibres of the peripheral nerve. The nociceptive conditioning stimuli used most probably involved $A\delta$ and C fiber nociceptive afferents. This seems particularly likely for the thermal conditioning stimuli since

Reflex   Sensation

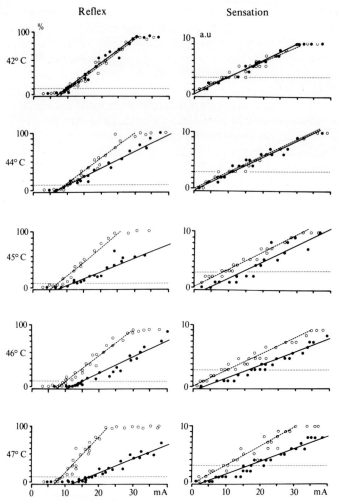

Fig. 5. Individual examples showing the effects of various conditioning thermal stimuli applied to the contralateral hand (temperatures indicated on the *left*) on the nociceptive reflex activity *(left)* and the corresponding subjective sensation *(right)* induced by sural nerve stimulation (*a.u.*, arbitrary units). For each sequence, control *(open circle, dotted line)* and conditioned *(filled circle, solid line)* recruitment curves are plotted on the same graph [146]

40°–44°C stimuli were ineffective whereas inhibitory effects were found between 45° and 47.5°C in a direct relationship with the temperature. In man, the pain threshold for thermal stimulation is achieved when skin temperature reaches approximately 45°C, [62], and pain scaling is possible only in the 44°–50°C range [1, 75]. In addition, pain scaling has been shown to be correlated with the firing of polymodal nociceptors during thermal noxious stimulation [2, 58]. Taken together, these data suggest that the observed inhibition induced by heterotopic thermal conditioning stimuli parallels both the sensation of pain and the responses of peripheral nociceptors.

86

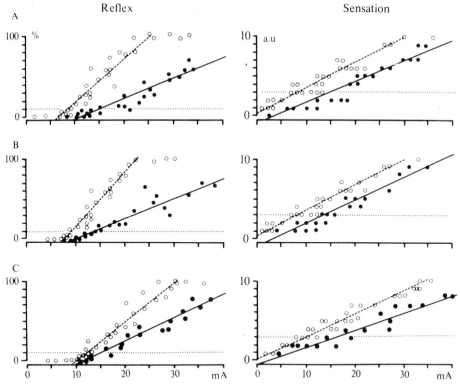

Fig. 6. Individual examples showing the effects of three heterotopic nociceptive conditioning stimuli (presentation and symbols as in Fig. 9). **A** Immersion of the left hand in an agitated waterbath maintained at 6 °C. **B** 10 watts muscular exercise with the left forearm during an ischemic block of arterial blood flow achieved using a pneumatic cuff placed around the middle part of the left arm and inflated to 1.5 times the systolic blood pressure. **C** Application of a pair of forceps (15–20 mm², 4.5 kg/cm²) to the nasal septum [146]

In a more recent study [147], the inhibitory effects of acute pain produced by the Lasègue's maneuver on the RIII reflex were explored in patients complaining of sciatica as a result of an identified unilateral disc protrusion. Lasègue's maneuver on the affected side produced a typical radicular pain and resulted in a powerful depression of nociceptive reflexes elicited either in the normal or in the affected lower limb. Simultaneously, patients reported relief of the electrically induced pain. In contrast, painless Lasègue's maneuver on the normal side had no effect on these parameters.

Thus, our data show that whether clinical or experimental and, in the latter case, whether induced by heat, cold, mechanical, or chemical procedures a painful conditioning stimulus strongly depresses, at spinal level, the nociceptive messages elicited from remote localized body areas. The site of application of the effective conditioning nociceptive stimuli could be far from the site of origin or the conditioned pain response, thus excluding segmental mechanisms or the involvement of trigger points [124].

The close relationship between the effects of the conditioning stimuli on the reflex and on the related sensation argues against a mechanism of inhibition acting on the motoneural pool. Instead, such a relationship suggests that these inhibitory mechanisms modulate a common spinal interneuronal pool responsible for both the nociceptive reflex and ascending pain pathways. The question arises as to the identity of the pathways mediating such inhibitory mechanism and, more particularly, whether they are confined to the spinal cord or whether they extend to supraspinal structures.

Involvement of Supraspinal Structures

In order to assess the possible involvement of supraspinal structures in these effects, we compared the effects of nociceptive electrical stimuli applied to the 4th and 5th fingers of the hand upon the contralateral RIII reflex in normal subjects and tetraplegic patients suffering from a clinically complete spinal cord section of traumatic origin [114].

In both groups, the RIII reflex threshold was determined, and a juxtathreshold RIII reflex was studied before, during, and after a 2-min period of conditioning stimulation. The nociceptive conditioning procedure consisted of electrical stimulation (1-ms duration pulses at 3 Hz) applied to the digital branches of the contralateral ulnar nerve which arises from C8 and T1. The intensity was adjusted to the maximum that normal subjects could tolerate (25–30 mA).

In normal subjects, the nociceptive electrical stimulation of the fingers induced rhythmic painful sensations described as being like a pin prick with additional burning and squeezing sensations originating from deep structures. As illustrated with an individual example in Fig. 7A, the conditioning stimuli induced a strong inhibition of the RIII reflex. This inhibition occurred rapidly within the first minute, lasted throughout the conditioning period and only gradually recovered during the following 5 min. By contrast, non-nociceptive electrical stimulation (0.1-ms duration, 6–8 mA, 3 Hz) of the fingers induced a rhythmic tactile sensation, and this type of conditioning stimulation produced no significant change in the RIII reflex.

The tetraplegic patients had a C5, C6, or C7 spinal cord section with the lower segments, notably C8 and T1 from which the digital branches of the ulnar nerve project, clinically uninjured. In these patients, sural nerve stimulation induced a biceps femoris reflex which did not differ from the RIII reflex recorded in normal subjects, either in terms of latency or of threshold. As illustrated by the example in Fig. 7B, the nociceptive conditioning stimulation did not produce any depression of the RIII reflex in these patients.

These results show that the effects of heterotopic nociceptive stimulation observed in normal humans are probably mediated by a complex loop involving supraspinal structures.

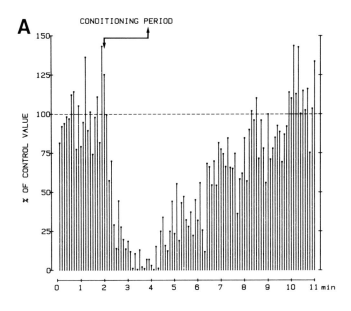

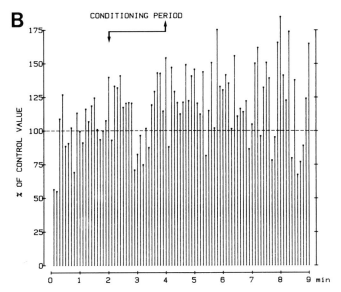

Fig. 7 A, B. Individual examples of the effects of heterotopic nociceptive stimulation upon the RIII reflex in a normal subject (**A**) and a tetraplegic patient (**B**). Each *bar* represents a single reflex response expressed as a percentage of the control level (0–2 min); the conditioning periods are indicated by *arrows* [114]

Involvement of the Brain Stem

This assertion is strongly supported by further unpublished experiments performed with brain-damaged patients involving analgesia and thermal anesthesia
on one side of the body. The lesions were located either in the parietal cortex or in
the thalamus (unilateral thalamic lesions visible on CT scanner) or in the retro-
olivary portion of the medulla (Wallenberg's syndrome).

With an experimental procedure identical to that reported above, the results
were unambiguous. In the case of parietal or thalamic lesions, the RIII reflex
recorded from the normal lower limb was strongly depressed by the nociceptive
but painless conditioning stimulation applied to the 4th and 5th fingers of the
affected hand. Inhibitory and poststimulus effects were identical to those observed
in normal subjects.

By contrast, in patients with Wallenberg's syndrome, e. g., in cases in which the
fibers originating from the anterolateral tract (including the spinothalamic, spinoreticular, and spinotectal tracts) were interrupted in the medulla, no signs of inhibition were detected when the affected hand was stimulated; when the contralateral, nonaffected hand was stimulated, inhibitory and poststimulus effects were
found, akin to those of normal subjects. These experiments demonstrate that
thalamic and suprathalamic structures are not involved in the inhibitory processes
described herein; whereas brain stem, probably reticular structures constitute a
key neuronal link in producing these effects.

Involvement of an Opioidergic Link

We reffered above to the possible involvement in animals of opioidergic systems
in hypoalgesia induced by a distant painful focus. In order to assess such an hypothesis in humans, we checked the effects of naloxone upon the electrophysiological model described above.

The RIII reflex threshold was determined, and a juxtathreshold RIII reflex was
studied before, during, and after a 2-min period of heterotopic conditioning stimulation (immersion of the contralateral hand in a 46.5 °C waterbath). As shown in
Fig. 8 with an individual example, such a manipulation resulted in a strong inhibition of the RIII reflex both during and after the conditioning period. Then, using
a double-blind paradigm, either saline or naloxone were injected IV. The results
were unambiguous in the nine normal volunteers tested in this way: while the
inhibitory effects could be repeated following saline injection, they disappeared
completely following naloxone administration (Fig. 8). Fifty minutes later the
inhibitory effects were observed in both cases, a finding which is consistent with
the well-known, short-acting action of the opioid antagonist.

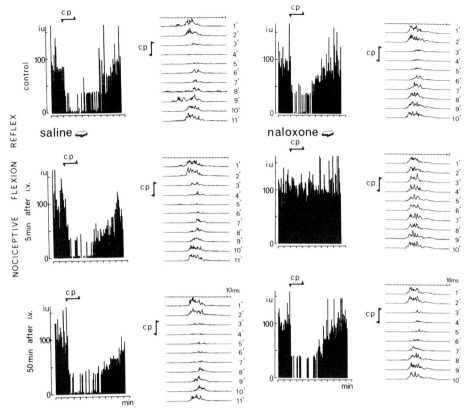

Fig. 8. Individual example showing the effect of a painful thermal stimulus (46 °C), applied for 2 min *(cp)* to the contralateral hand, on the RIII reflex before *(control)*, 5 min and 50 min after IV administration of saline *(left)* and of naloxone *(right)*. In each case, data are presented both as histograms *(left)* and as averaged responses *(right)*. Note the lack of inhibition of the RIII reflex 5 min after naloxone, but it is observed again 50 min after injection

Electrophysiological Approach in Animals

Diffuse Noxious Inhibitory Controls (DNIC)

In the rat, the activity of certain dorsal horn neurons can be strongly inhibited by noxious inputs. Since such effects do not appear to be somatotopically organized but do concern the entire body, they have been called diffuse noxious inhibitory controls (DNIC) [77, 78]. DNIC affect the whole population of convergent neurons, whether recorded in the superficial or deeper layers within the dorsal horn of various segments of the spinal cord [20, 77] or in the trigeminal nucleus caudalis [37]. By contrast, DNIC do not affect the other neuronal types that are found within the dorsal horn or nucleus caudalis, i.g., noxious specific, nonnoxious specific, cold responsive, and proprioceptive neurons [37, 78]. Recently, the existence of DNIC has been demonstrated in the cat [104].

91

The main feature of DNIC is that they can be triggered from any part of the body, distant from the excitatory receptive field of the neuron under study provided that this conditioning stimulus is clearly noxious. Indeed, DNIC can be triggered by any heterotopic nociceptive stimulus whatever its type – mechanical, thermal, chemical, or electrical – whereas nonnoxious stimuli are completely ineffective. For strong stimuli, the inhibitory effects are powerful and followed by long-lasting after effects which can persist for several minutes.

When the general characteristics of DNIC are analyzed, one striking feature is their capacity to affect all kinds of activities of convergent neurons, whether evoked from the periphery by noxious or nonnoxious, natural or electrical stimuli or directly by the microelectrophoretic application of excitatory aminoacids [132, 133]. Transcutaneous electrical stimuli applied to the receptive field or convergent neurons produce an activation of large (A) and fine (C) fibers, and in systematic studies of DNIC, suprathreshold currents have been employed in this way, to evoke a reproducible "C-fiber response" from convergent neurons. All noxious conditioning stimuli tested have induced marked inhibitions of these responses. Both the strength and long duration of DNIC are illustrated in Fig. 9, in which the response of a convergent neuron to a pinch applied on its receptive field is conditioned by various distant noxious stimuli.

It has been shown that the spinothalamic tract contains numerous convergent neurons; since nearly all convergent neurons tested have been influenced by DNIC, one can assume that DNIC will influence the transmission of information from convergent neurons to the brain. This assertion has been verified in the rat [36] by demonstrating that DNIC affect identified spinothalamic and trigeminothalamic convergent neurons.

The studies cited so far involved the use of acute stimuli, and it seemed essential to investigate also the way in which DNIC act in situations more relevant to clinical pain. Rats rendered arthritic by intradermal injection of Frend's adjuvant into the tail are considered to be a model of chronic pain relevant to human rheumatoid arthritis [31, 34, 111]. We chose to record dorsal horn neurons between the third and the fourth week following the adjuvant inoculation since in a recent study [21] it was found that such a period was critical for this disease in terms of both clinical, including radiological, observations and behavioral data, including pain-related tests.

As facial areas are not affected by arthritis, we recorded from trigeminal nucleus caudalis neurons in order to investigate the effects of heterotopically applied stimuli of various intensities on the responses of convergent neurons whose receptive fields were not in regions affected by the disease [23]. All convergent neurons were inhibited by heterotopic stimuli, whether noxious (52 °C, pinch) or nonnoxious (light and mild pressure), applied to inflamed areas. While the inhibitions triggered by noxious stimuli were similar to those observed in healthy rats, those triggered by nonnoxious mechanical stimuli had never previously been found when such stimuli were applied heterotopically in healthy animals. Moreover, the strength of these inhibitions was related to the inflammatory state of the part of the body stimulated, the most sensitive areas being the hind paws; in this case, light and mild pressure resulted in 60% and 100% inhibition, respectively, followed by long-lasting after effects (several minutes).

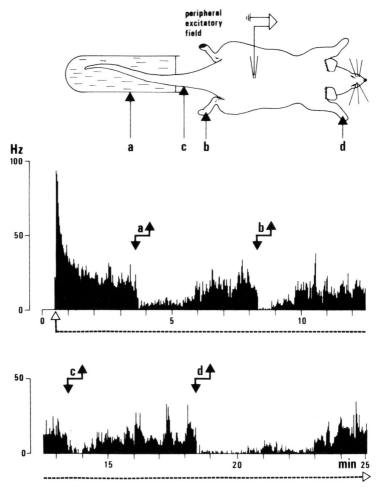

Fig. 9. Inhibitory effects induced by various heterotopic noxious stimuli upon the response of a convergent neuron to a sustained pinch [18]. The application of a sustained pinch *(open arrowhead, broken line)* to the peripheral excitatory field of the lumbar convergent neuron located on the hind paw extremity resulted in a phasic response followed by a tonic discharge. Various stimuli *(solid arrowheads)* induced strong inhibitory effects followed by long-lasting after effects: *a,* immersion of the tail in a 52 °C water bath; *b,* pinch of the contralateral hind paw; *c,* pinch of the tail; *d,* pinch of a forepaw

The increase in peripheral sensitivity induced by arthritis could account for such an augmentation of the heterotopic inhibitory phenomena. Peripheral changes induced by arthritis have been described: joint capsule receptors, which have nonmyelinated or poorly myelinated axons, have lower thresholds to mechanical stimulation [57], and some dorsal horn neurons exhibit exaggerated responses to light mechanical stimulation [22, 100].

DNIC cannot be demonstrated in anesthetized or decerebrate animals in which the spinal cord has been sectioned [18, 78, 104]. Therefore, the mechanisms underlying DNIC are obviously not confined to the spinal cord, and thus supraspinal structures must be implicated in the circuits. In this respect, it is important to note that such a system is completely different from segmental inhibitory systems since segmental inhibitory receptive fields are found in both intact and spinal animals. Furthermore, this latter type of inhibition can be triggered by the activation of low threshold afferents. DNIC are also completely different from propriospinal inhibitory processes triggered by noxious inputs [18, 45, 51].

Peripheral Mechanisms

The correlation between the intensity of a noxious stimulus and the resultant strength of DNIC would seem to be an important point to investigate. For simplicity and technical ease, we considered the effect of various temperatures applied to the tail on the C-fiber responses of lumbar and trigeminal convergent neurons elicited by transcutaneous electrical stimulation of their hind paw or facial receptive fields [79, 131]. As shown in Fig. 10, the threshold for producing DNIC is between 40° and 44 °C, and above this temperature (in the range 44°–52 °C), a highly significant correlation exists between the conditioning temperature and the degree of inhibition. In addition, analogous results have been obtained when identical thermal stimuli were tested against activities evoked by microelectrophoresis of an excitatory amino acid [131].

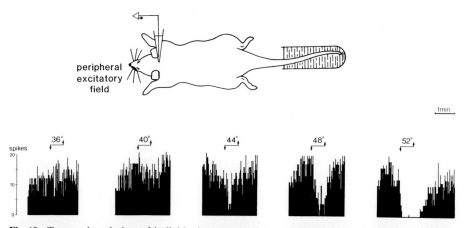

Fig. 10. Temporal evolution of individual responses due to C-fiber inputs of a nucleus caudalis convergent neuron before, during, and after the application of various temperatures to the tail. Each *histogram* represents the temporal evolution *(abscissa,* time) of the responses due to C-fibers *(ordinate,* number of spikes in the 50–120 ms period following the stimulus) when transcutaneous electrical stimuli (2 ms 12 mA, 0.66 Hz) were applied in the center of the excitatory receptive field. From the 45th to the 70th stimulus *(arrows),* the distal two-thirds of the tail were immersed in a waterbath at various temperatures (indicated *between arrows*). Note that nonnociceptive temperatures 36°, 40 °C) did not affect the neuronal discharges. At 44 °C discrete inhibitory effects occurred; these increased as the temperature increased [131]

These data reinforce the hypothesis that DNIC are triggered specifically by the activation of peripheral nociceptors whose signals are carried by Aδ- and C-fibers. C polymodal nociceptors have been described in the cat, rat, monkey, rabbit, and humans [131]. They constitute a large proportion of the total population of C-fiber afferents in these species, and it is important to note that, to date, all C-fibers recorded in humans have shown the characteristics of polymodal nociceptors [123, 130]. In addition, a population of Aδ myelinated polymodal nociceptors responding to thermal stimuli exists, and these have electrophysiological characteristics essentially similar to those of C polymodal nociceptors; they have been described in monkeys and humans [131]. Both types of polymodal nociceptors increase their discharges when the temperatures applied to their receptive fields increase, especially in the 45°–51°C range. According to Lamotte and Campbell [75] their mean threshold for activation is 43.6°C. Finally, Dubner and Beitel [41] have reported a good correlation between the activity of polymodal nociceptors triggered by thermal stimulation and escape behavior in the monkey. This strongly suggests that DNIC are specifically triggered by the activation of nociceptors.

We then investigated the types of peripheral fibers involved in DNIC [14]. For this purpose, we took advantage of the facts that trigeminal and spinal dorsal horn neurons respond with relatively steady discharges to the electrophoretic application of excitatory amino-acids and that DNIC act on convergent neurons by a final postsynaptic inhibitory mechanism involving hyperpolarization of the neuronal membrane [132, 133]. It was found that when trigeminal convergent neurons were directly excited by the electrophoretic application of dl-homocysteate (DLH), the percutaneous electrical application of single square-wave stimuli (10 mA; 2 ms) to the tail always induced a biphasic depression of such activity. Both the early and late components of this inhibition occurred with shorter latencies when the base rather than the tip of the tail was stimulated (Fig. 11). Since the two stimulation sites were 100 mm apart, it was possible to use these differences in latencies from the two sites to estimate the conduction velocities of the peripheral fibers triggering the inhibitions. For the onset of the earlier and later components of the inhibition, the mean differences between the latencies from the two sites of stimulation were 13.6 and 147.7 ms, respectively, corresponding to peripheral conduction velocities of 7.3 and 0.68 m/s respectively. According to Gasser and Erlanger [50] and Burgess and Perl [17], these values correspond to peripheral conduction velocities in the Aδ- and C-fiber ranges, respectively.

Although peripheral unmyelinated and thin myelinated fibers can respond to stimuli below the pain threshold [2, 58, 123, 129], the relationship between the activation of such fibers and nociceptive reactions or pain is a classical one [2, 41, 58, 75, 123, 129]. However, the thresholds for triggering the Aδ- and C-fiber components were found to be in the 0.25–0.5 mA and 1–2 mA ranges, respectively, which could be interpreted as suggesting a possible contribution by nonnociceptive afferents.

The importance of Aδ-fiber activation in the production of analgesia or antinociceptive effects by somatic electrical stimulation has been suggested by several authors [29, 69, 85, 120, 149]. In this respect, our results showed that, by comparison with the C-fiber component, the Aδ-fiber component of inhibition was easier to obtain and more constant in terms of magnitude and duration: it was observed

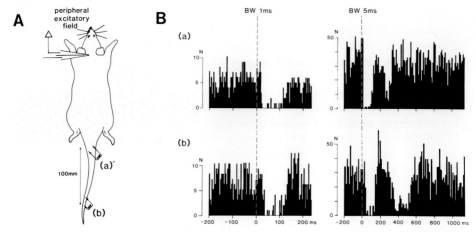

Fig. 11 A, B. Example of the heterotopic activation of Aδ- and C-fibers triggering inhibition of a trigeminal convergent neuron [14]. **A** Schematic representation of the experimental design. Neurons with receptive fields located ipsilaterally on the muzzle were recorded at the trigeminal nucleus caudalis. The continuous electrophoretic application of an excitatory amino acid, dl-homocysteic acid (DLH), induced a steady discharge from the neuron under study. The repetitive application of individual percutaneous, electrical stimuli of adequate intensities to the base *(a)* or the tip *(b)* of the tail induced biphasic depressions of activity which exclusively affected convergent neurons. **B** Individual example of the biphasic inhibitory processes triggered by repetitive, single, percutaneous, electrical stimuli (2 ms duration, 10 mA, 0.66 Hz, 200 ms delay) applied to the base **(a)** or the tip **(b)** of the tail on the discharge of a trigeminal convergent neuron, evoked by the continuous electrophoretic application of DLH (17 nA). Peristimulus histograms (bin width: 1 ms *left;* 5 ms, *right*) were constructed from 100 trials. The earlier component of the inhibition is detailed in the *left part* of the figure while the whole biphasic inhibition is shown on the *right*. Note that both components appeared earlier when the base **(a)** as opposed to the tip **(b)** of the tail was stimulated

with lower intensities of percutaneous electrical stimulation and rapidly reached its maximum effect when the current was increased. Applying stronger intensities of peripheral stimuli gave rise to inhibitory effects of similar magnitude. This difference between the Aδ- and C-fiber components is probably due to the fact that, in addition to having lower threshold, the Aδ-fibers responsible for the earlier inhibitions produce a more synchronized input to the spinal cord than do the slower C-fibers. The "safety" of the Aδ-fiber component of inhibition is also illustrated in Fig. 12, in which currents of 1 mA were applied percutaneously to the base of the tail at different frequencies. Such an intensity was chosen because it was found to induce clear Aδ- but no C-fiber components of inhibition. Note that the inhibitory processes followed increasing frequencies of stimulation, although they were slightly less effective with the highest frequency employed (8 Hz). This observation reinforces the proposal that Aδ-fibers play an important role in the induction of analgesia or hypoalgesia by procedures using transcutaneous stimulation, since such procedures often involve these frequencies of stimulation (see below).

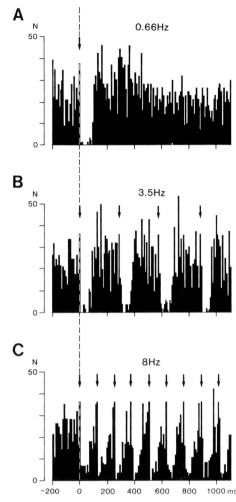

Fig. 12 A–C. Individual example of the inhibitory effects induced by percutaneous electrical stimuli (2 ms duration, 1 mA, 200 ms delay) applied at different frequencies to the base of the tail, on the DLH-evoked activity (15 nA) of a trigeminal convergent neuron. Peristimulus histograms (bin width 5 ms) were composed from 100 trials. Note that the A component presents the same magnitude when frequencies of 0.66 and 3.5 Hz were applied, whereas it decreased slightly with the highest frequency employed (8 Hz) [14]

Involvement of the Anterolateral Quadrant

We have already mentioned that DNIC acting on convergent lumbar neurones are abolished by total section of the (cervical) spinal cord. It appears, therefore, that the involvement of a supraspinal loop is essential for the triggering of DNIC. In order to determine the anatomical profile of the ascending limb of the loop subserving DNIC, we made use of the fact that DNIC act on nucleus caudalis convergent neurons. By triggering DNIC from a caudal region of the body, we were able to study a model in which the circuitry of the loop consisted of a long ascend-

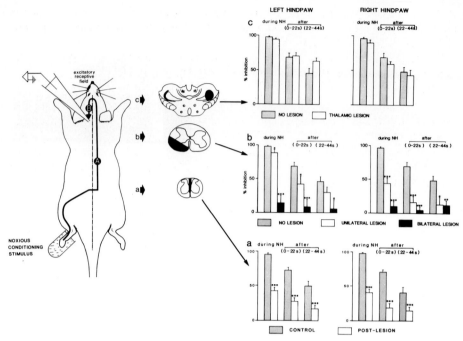

Fig. 13a–c. Ascending pathways involved in the triggering of DNIC [134]. *Left,* schematic representation of the experimental design. Convergent neurons with receptive fields located ipsilaterally on the muzzle were recorded in the left trigeminal nucleus caudalis. C-fiber responses were conditioned by immersion of either hindpaw in a 52 °C water bath. With this experimental arrangement the supraspinal loop sustaining DNIC comprised a long ascending *(A)* and a short descending *(B)* pathway. The effects of three types of CNS lesions were studied: **a** lumbar commissurotomy, **b** cervical sections, and **c** destruction of the right ventrobasal thalamic complex. *Right,* summary of results. *Histograms* represent the percentage inhibitions observed during *(during NH)* and within the 44 s after *(after 0–22 s, after 22–44 s)* the immersion of the left *(left histograms)* or the right *(right histograms)* hind paws. Controls are shown as *hatched bars.* **a** Lumbar commissurotomy: Note the symmetrical nature of the reductions of the inhibitions triggered from either hind paw which were induced by the commissurotomy *(open bars)*. **b** Anterolateral lesions: Inhibitions observed in rats with unilateral *(open bars)* or bilateral lesions *(solid bars)* are compared with those observed in untransected animals. Note that in unilateral lesions, inhibitory processes triggered from the right hind paw were strongly reduced, with the poststimulus effects disappearing almost completely while inhibitory processes triggered from the left hind paw were slightly decreased. Also, in bilateral lesions, the inhibitions, whether triggered from the left or the right hind paw, disappeared almost completely. **c** Lesion of the right ventrobasal thalamic complex. Note that the inibitions could be triggered equally from either hind paw *(open bars)* and that they did not differ significantly from those observed in intact rats

ing (Fig. 13 a) and a short descending (Fig. 13 b) pathway [134]. In such a situation, a blockade of DNIC by subtotal spinal section would have to be due to the inpairment of nociceptive transmission in the ascending spinal pathways rather than of transmission in descending pathways to the trigeminal system. The use of a thermal nociceptive conditioning stimulus applied to either the left or right hindpaw allowed us to compare the strength of DNIC before and following: lumbar commissurotomy (Fig. 13 a), restricted lesions of the cervical spinal cord corresponding to various sensory ascending pathways, unilateral and bilateral sections of the anterolateral quadrant at the cervical level (Fig. 13 b), and thalamic lesions (Fig. 13 c).

Two ascertain the possible crossed nature of the pathways responsible for the heterotopic processes, the effects of lumbar commissurotomy were investigated. As shown in Fig. 13 a, the inhibitory processes, whether triggered from the left or right hindpaw, were strongly depressed in all the experiments. However, this depression was not complete, suggesting that both crossed and uncrossed components play a role.

Lesioning dorsal, dorsolateral, and ventromedial parts of the cervical cord was found not to affect inhibitory processes triggered from either hindpaw. It appeared therefore that several sensory pathways for which roles in nociception have been suggested could not have been involved, namely: the postsynaptic fibers of the dorsal columns [7, 8, 52, 55, 128], the spinocervical tract which travels through the dorsolateral funiculus [32, 53, 90, 103], and part of the spinothalamic tract, i.e., those fibers projecting to the medial and intralaminar thalamus and travelling through the ventromedial funiculus [53].

On the other hand, our results strongly indicate that there is an essential role for the anterolateral quadrant in the triggering of DNIC, since it was this region alone that remained undamaged when the overlap of the lesions that were unable to attenuate DNIC was considered. Conversely, all the lesions that reduced DNIC triggered from the hindpaw included the anterolateral region of the opposite side or at least the lateral part of that region.

Furthermore, unilateral lesions of the left anterolateral quadrant resulted in a strong reduction of inhibitory processes triggered from the right hindpaw, whereas the inhibition triggered from the left hindpaw was slightly, albeit significantly, decreased (Fig. 13 b, *open bars*). Bilateral lesions of the anterolateral quadrant resulted in a complete disappearance of inhibitions, whether triggered from the right or the left hindpaw (Fig. 13 b, *solid bars*). Thus, the lateral spinothalamic tract [13, 53, 54, 70, 93] and the part of the spinoreticular system which travels within the anterolateral quadrant [92, 93, 150] could have been involved.

The mainly crossed nature of the ascending pathways subserving DNIC suggests the participation of spinothalamic neurons in these processes. It has been shown in the rat that ascending projections reaching the lateral thalamus are completely crossed [109], and the axons of spinothalamic neurons are classically described as crossing the midline at the level of the segment containing the cell body [46, 148]. All these considerations prompted us to undertake the last series of experiments in which the neurons of the right lateral thalamus were destroyed by prior microinjection of kainic acid. The results were unambiguous: DNIC were triggered equally well from either hindpaw after large lesions involving the right ventrobasal thalamic complex (Fig. 13 c). These experiments therefore eliminated a possible lateral thalamic link in the loop subserving DNIC.

The remaining candidate for a role in triggering DNIC is the spinoreticular tract, since it has been clearly established that the axons of this tract are located in the anterolateral region of the spinal cord [70, 92, 93]. Interestingly, in the rat these pathways have been shown to have a crossed and an uncrossed component [92, 93, 150].

Involvement of Nucleus Raphe Magnus

Due to the ascending/descending nature of the inhibitory loop originating from the peripheral nociceptors, it is tempting to speculate that DNIC involve certain of those brain structures, the electrical stimulation of which can depress the activities of convergent neurons [10]. In the rat for instance, stimulation of nucleus raphe magnus (NRM) powerfully inhibits the responses of convergent neurons [112] to a degree comparable with that produced by DNIC. We have therefore directly investigated its involvement in DNIC by comparing the inhibitory effects of DNIC on trigeminal nucleus caudalis and dorsal horn convergent neurons before and after electrolytic lesions of the NRM [38]. In most neurons recorded in a group of rats in which the cumulative lesions destroyed areas of the brain stem including the NRM, the ventral part of the nucleus reticularis paragigantocellularis (NRPG), and the midline reticular formation immediately dorsal to the NRM, a strong reduction of DNIC was apparent, both immediately after the lesion and also in later tests. Due to the difficulty of confining lesions to the NRM, we cannot rule out a participation of the medial part of the NRPG in some of these effects. Interestingly, this medial area and the region of the NRPG overlying the pyramidal tract also contain serotonergic cell bodies, and these areas together with NRM coincide with nucleus B3 of Dahlstrom and Fuxe [33], in their original description of serotonergic cell areas.

Involvement of a Serotonergic Link

Considering that the NRM is rich in serotonin-containing cell bodies, and since serotonin (5-HT) plays a major role in descending control systems [76], the effects of various manipulations of serotonergic systems on DNIC were studied. These included the depletion of 5-HT by para-chlorophenylalanine (PCPA), blockade of 5-HT receptors, and administration of the precursor of 5-HT, 5-hydroxytryptophan (5-HTP).

Pretreatment with PCPA (300 mg/kg, IP, 3 days) resulted in a strong reduction in DNIC [39]; the after effects were also reduced in terms of their magnitude and duration. It is worth pointing out that although our pretreatment procedure induced a total 5-HT depletion at the spinal level, the blockade of DNIC was not complete. This observation suggests that additional nonserotonergic mechanisms are involved in DNIC.

The results presented above needed further confirmation since the effect of PCPA is not totally restricted to 5-HT depletion. We therefore utilized complementary pharmacological tools, e.g., 5-HT receptor blockers (cinanserin and metergoline) and a precursor of 5-HT synthesis. Both systemic cinancerin and metergoline strongly reduced DNIC, whereas 5-HTP increased the inhibitory effects [28].

The most likely site of action for the effects we have reported with systemically administered drugs is on serotonergic, bulbospinal, descending inhibitory pathways. However, it may be noted that we cannot rule out the possibility that the effects reported above may have involved serotonergic systems other than the bulbospinal pathways.

The idea of descending serotonergic pathways being activated by noxious stimuli is supported by biochemical lines of evidence. It has been shown that bilateral high intensity – but not low intensity – stimulation of the sciatic nerve induces a release of 5-HT in superfusates from the spinal cord of the cat; thoracic cold block prevents this effect [127]. Since a rise in 5-HT release was also observed following stimulation of the infraorbital branch of the trigeminal nerve, it is possible to suggest that there is a diffuse release of the monoamine within the cord no matter what part of the body is stimulated; interestingly, 5-HT release can be induced by electrical stimulation of the DLF [127], the NRM, or the NRPG [59, 110, 113]. In addition, the prolonged application of intense nociceptive electrical stimuli to the tail of anesthetized rats induced a rise in 5-HT synthesis in the dorsal part of the cord: by contrast, the prolonged application of innocuous electrical stimuli to the tail was not followed by any detectable change in 5-HT synthesis [140]. Furthermore, electrical stimulation of the NRM has also been reported to produce increased synthesis of 5-HT within the cord [12].

Involvement of an Opioidergic Link

The parallels between both types of inhibition (NRM- and DNIC-mediated) are further emphasized by the fact that both are decreased to a comparable extent by the opioid antagonist naloxone, at least in the rat and when experiments are performed under identical conditions. Indeed, comparison of the results related to DNIC in the rat [80] with those of Rivot et al. [112] for NRM stimulation in the same species, shows that the antagonistic effect of systemic naloxone was of the same magnitude for DNIC- and NRM-mediated inhibitions.

As we have used only systemic injections of naloxone, we have no way of knowing the location of its action. However, two distinct hypotheses might be advanced, based on the anatomical localization of opioidergic interneurons: naloxone could antagonize DNIC at supraspinal and/or at spinal sites. No matter which of these is correct, as it is generally agreed that naloxone is a pure opiate antagonist – at least in low doses – the data therefore strongly suggest a participation of endogenous opioids in DNIC.

The possible participation of spinal opioids in DNIC is supported by biochemical data showing that a noxious mechanical stimulus does not alter the release of met-enkephalin-like material (MELM) from neuronal segments related to the stimulated area of the body but does increase its release from other segments [83]. Interestingly, in an additional study, we demonstrated that this heterosegmental release of MELM is sustained by activity in descending pathways travelling in the DLF [84]. This probably implies that the release of MELM is sustained by a supraspinal loop since a large number of studies have implicated the DLF as the descending part of an inhibitory system originating from the brain stem (see above).

Involvement of the Dorsolateral Funiculus

To analyze the anatomical profile of the descending tracts of the loop subserving DNIC, inhibitions were triggered from a rostral part of the body, and recordings were made from lumbar dorsal horn convergent neurons [135]. In this situation the

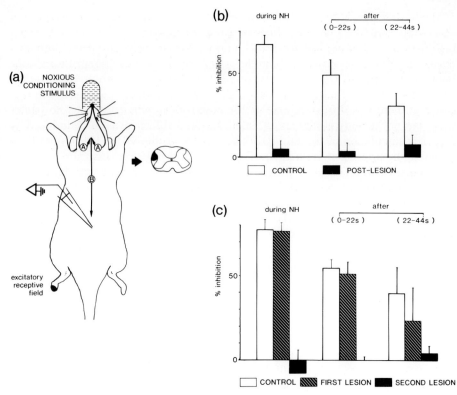

Fig. 14 a-c. Involvement of the dorsolateral funiculus (DLF) in the triggering of diffuse noxious inhibitory controls (DNIC) [135]. **a** Schematic representation of the experimental design. Convergent neurons with receptive field located on the extremity of the ipsilateral hind paw were recorded in the dorsal horn of the lumbar spinal cord. C-fiber responses were conditioned by immersion of the muzzle in a 52 °C water bath. With this experimental arrangement, the loop sustaining DNIC comprised a short ascending *(A)* and a long descending *(B)* pathway. Effects of restricted cervical lesions involving the DLF were studied. **b** Summary of experiments involving a single ipsilateral DLF lesion. *Histograms* represent the percentage inhibition observed during *(during NH)* and within the 44 s following *(after 0-22 s, after 22-44 s)* the immersion of the muzzle in a 52 °C water bath. Note that the inhibitory processes *(open bars)* disappeared after the DLF lesions *(solid bars).* **c** Summary of the experiments involving two consecutive DLF lesions. Note that inhibitory processes were not essentially different before *(open bars)* and after *(hatched bars)* contralateral DLF lesions. In contrast, after ipsilateral DLF lesions *(solid bars)* the inhibitory processes were abolished

circuitry of the loop involves a short ascending (Fig. 14a) and a long descending (Fig. 14b) pathway. In such a situation, blockade of DNIC by a subtotal spinal section would have to be due to the impairment of transmission in the descending part of the loop. A thermal nociceptive conditioning stimulus (52 °C) applied to the muzzle allowed us to compare the strength of DNIC before and after lesions of the dorsolateral part of the cervical spinal cord. Such an experimental design was chosen in an attempt to answer the question of whether the ipsilateral and/or contralateral DLF to the recording site carries signals responsible for DNIC.

As shown in Fig. 14b, a lesion which included the DLF ipsilateral to the neuron under study completely abolished the inhibitory processes triggered from the muzzle. In order to confirm that the descending projections responsible for DNIC lie mainly if not exclusively in the ipsilateral DLF, the effects of a lesion of the contralateral DLF were investigated. Neither the inhibitory processes nor the unconditioned C-fiber responses were altered by this procedure; however, a second lesion including the ipsilateral DLF again induced a blockade of DNIC (Fig. 14c).

One can therefore conclude that the descending projections involved in the triggering of DNIC are mainly, if not entirely, confined to the DLF ipsilateral to the neuron under study.

The relationship between the DLF and the descending serotonergic systems was first established by the work of Dahlstrom and Fuxe [33], who found that in the rat 5-HT-containing axons descending through the lateral funiculi project to the superficial layers of the spinal cord. Skagerberg and Bjorklund [121] showed that most of the 5-HT-containing axons originating from the brain stem and with spinal projections descend ipsilaterally in the DLF, whereas the descending, non-5-HT projections present a bilateral funicular distribution. In this respect, we have already referred to evidence for the participation of 5-HT in DNIC.

Counterirritation and the Alleviation of Pain by Percutaneous Electrical Stimulation and Acupuncture

There have been numerous studies concerning analgesia produced by TENS in humans [4]. Although it can often be explained by the inhibitory processes triggered by $A\alpha$ and β receptors input at the segmental level [96, 106, 136], the conclusions from human experiments and the mechanisms underlying TENS and electroacupuncture applied to sites with or without segmental relation to the pain locus require an explanation based on several mechanisms [5, 6, 44, 67, 95, 105, 116]. In this respect, it is important to point out that the proposed gate control theory [96] is mainly focused on segmental spinal inhibitory mechanisms, and therefore the pain-alleviating effects of remote stimulation require a different functional basis.

Although TENS can be effective when applied at high frequencies and intensities below the pain threshold (see Fig. 15), the resulting pain relief is more localized and often limited to the stimulated segment [4]. Furthermore, it has also been shown that stronger analgesic effects can be obtained with TENS by using a critical level of stimulation which produces an unpleasant but not quite painful sensation [4]. Finally, it has been shown in primates that TENS inhibits C-fibers-evoked responses of spinothalamic tract cells only when the intensity of TENS exceeds the threshold for activating $A\delta$-fibers [85].

Analgesic effects produced by electroacupuncture or acupuncture often employ intensities of stimulation strong enough to induce the feeling of 'De Qi', an unpleasant sensation reminiscent of pain [17]: this procedure results in pain relief with a widespread distribution. We have proposed [78] that DNIC may well form the neural basis of the pain-relieving effects of such procedures in which afferent $A\delta$ or $A\delta$ and C fibers play an important role (see above). It is therefore con-

103

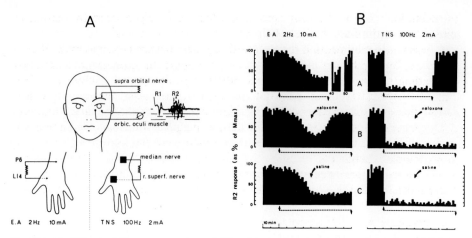

Fig. 15 A, B. Effects of electroacupuncture *(EA)* and transcutaneous nerve stimulation *(TNS)* on the nociceptive component of the blink reflex [144]. The blink reflex was elicited by electrical stimulation of the supraorbitary nerve at noxious intensity, and recordings were made from the orbicularis ocularis muscle [73, 142]. EA involved stimulation of the wrist via needle electrodes (square pulses of 0.5 ms duration, 10–12 mA intensity, 1–3 Hz) and homosegmental TNS was applied to the supraorbital nerve (square pulses of 0.2 ms, 2–4 mA intensity, 80–100 Hz). **A** Experimental procedure for eliciting and recording the R2 component of the blink reflex. **B** Individual example. R2 responses are expressed as percentage of the maximal control motor response *(M,* maximum). Note *left,* the progressive and moderate naloxone-sensitive depression in the R2 response obtained with EA; and *right,* the rapid and major depression in the R2 response which was not modified by naloxone

ceivable that, at least in some circumstances, TENS and electroacupuncture could share common mechanisms.

In other cases, this is clearly not the case as illustrated in Fig. 15 in which the nociceptive component (R2) of the blink reflex was recorded [144, 145]. Electroacupuncture applied to the wrist yielded a progressive decrease of the R2 response of the blink reflex, which was long lasting and naloxone sensitive. By contrast, the application of homosegmental TENS produced a very quick fall of the R2 reflex, which ceased as soon as TENS was stopped and was not affected by naloxone.

The assertion that, in some cases, analgesia elicited by acupuncture techniques may involve DNIC is strongly supported by results obtained from several Chinese workers, although the question of the specificity of the acupuncture points is rarely investigated. However, it has been reported that the analgesia produced is widespread and bilateral but with a greater segmental effect [26]. This later point may relate to the involvement of the large fibre mediated segmental effect in addition to a DNIC-mediated widespread effect. A description of the sensation of the acupuncture stimulation is also rarely given, but it seems that, in some cases, thin fibers are the origin of the analgesic effects observed. For instance, in man, vascular occlusion (lasting 20 min) applied to the upper arm does not affect the analgesic effect induced by the needling of points located below the level of occlusion [26]. Under these conditions, it is well-known that conduction is reduced primarily in large myelinated fibers with slowly conducting fibers being affected to a lesser extent. Furthermore, it has previously been reported that during an almost identical occlusion, pain is the only sensation which can be produced by peripheral stimulation of the occluded area [61].

A series of experiments [27, 40, 118] using electroacupuncture versus viscerosomatic reflex discharges in animals strongly supports the idea of the ascending-descending nature of the mechanisms subserving this kind of analgesia: inhibitions disappeared in spinal preparations but remained after decerebration, suggesting that the brain stem contains the main link in these phenomena. More precisely, a lesion of the median region of the medulla, principally including the NRM, produced a strong reduction of the inhibitory effects, which also, according to sectioning experiments, required the anterolateral and the dorsolateral funiculus as ascending and descending pathways, respectively. These results strongly suggest that both ascending pain pathways and descending inhibitory pathways are involved.

In addition, Han and Terenius [60] reviewed evidence for an important, if not prevalent, role for central serotonergic mechanisms in mediating acupuncture analgesia. The analogy between some forms of electroacupuncture and DNIC is also supported by the fact that in the spinal trigeminal nucleus, convergent units are inhibited by electroacupuncture whereas noxious – only units are unaffected [35]. This analogy is furthered by numerous data which have shown the involvement of endogenous opioid peptides, particularly at the brain stem level (NRM, PAG) in the mechanisms of acupuncture analgesia [65].

Finally, in a recent, unpublished study, we observed that the inhibitions of convergent neurons recorded within the spinal trigeminal nucleus were reduced to a similar extent by systemic naloxone, whether they were triggered by the immersion of a hind paw in a 50°C water bath or by the manual stimulation of the St. 36 Zusanli point on the tibialis anterior muscle.

Summary

We have provided electrophysiological evidence from both humans and animals that counterirritation phenomena have a well-defined, neural substrate explanation. Indeed, the following points appear to be common to the RIII reflex recorded in humans and convergent neurons recorded in rats:
1. The RIII reflex and the responses of convergent neurons to electrical stimulation of their receptive fields can be inhibited by various heterotopic noxious stimuli.
2. The distance between the conditioned and conditioning sites of stimulation is not a critical factor for the strength of the inhibitions.
3. All types of conditioning nociceptive stimuli, whether electrical, mechanical, thermal, or chemical, are effective.
4. The inhibitions are directly related to the strength of the conditioning stimuli.
5. They are powerful and affect responses to both threshold and suprathreshold electrical shocks.
6. They are followed by moderately long-lasting, after-stimulus effects.
7. In both cases, the inhibitions are enhanced in pathological situations (i.e., Lasegue maneuver in humans, arthritis in rats).

8. They require a complex loop ascending from and descending to the spinal cord.
9. In both cases, the loop does not involve spinothalamic fibers but includes brain stem structures and spinoreticular fibers.
10. There is an opioidergic link in the loop.
11. Finally, DNIC have been shown in the rat to affect both the responses of spino-thalamic convergent neurons [36] and the polysynaptic reflex discharges in the common peroneal nerve following electrical stimulation of the sural nerve [119]. These observations indicate the ability of DNIC to modulate nociceptive information transmitted by ascending pain pathways and also by nociceptive reflex pathways. Our psychophysical and neurophysiological experiments show that related events occur in humans.

These parallels lead us to believe that the inhibitory effects observed in humans and DNIC in rats share common mechanisms. These mechanisms are observed when two noxious stimuli are applied to distinct areas of the body, thus inducing a competitive effect. These effects, sustained by supraspinal structures and depressing the transmission of nociceptive messages at the spinal level, could have numerous neurological consequences. Further studies of the DNIC circuitry in humans could help to elucidate the role of descending controls both in normal and pathological situations.

Acknowledgements. This work was supported by l'Institut Nation de la Santé et de la Recherche Médicale (INSERM), la Direction des Recherches et Études Techniques (DRET), and La Fondation pour la Recherche Médicale. The authors are very grateful to Drs. Besson, Bouhassira, Bussel, Cadden, Calvino, Cesaro, Chaouch, Chitour, Dickenson, Kraus, Peschanski, Rivot, and Roby-Brami for their contribution to some aspects of this work, to Dr. Cadden for advice in the preparation of the manuscript, to Mrs. M. Gras for the typing, and to E. Dehausse and J. Chandellier for drawings and photography.

References

1. Adair EE, Stevens, JC, Marks LE (1968) Thermally induced pain: the dol scale and the psychological power law. Am J Psychol 81: 147–164
2. Adriansen H, Gybels J, Handwerker HO, Van Hees J (1983) Response properties of thin myelinated ($A\delta$) fibres in human skin nerves. J Neurophysiol 49: 111–122
3. Andersson KV, Pearl GS, Honeycutt C (1976) Behavioural evidence showing the predominance of diffuse pain stimuli over discrete stimuli in influencing perception. J Neurosci Res 2: 283–289
4. Andersson SA (1979) Pain control by sensory stimulation. In: Bonica JJ, Liebeskind JC, Albe-Fessard D (eds), Advances in pain research and therapy, vol 3. Raven, New York, pp 569–585
5. Andersson SA, Holmgren E (1975) On acupuncture analgesia and the mechanism of pain. Am J Chin Med 3: 311–334
6. Andersson SA, Holmgren E, Roos A (1977) Analgesic effects of peripheral conditioning stimulation: II. Importance of certain stimulation parameters. Acupunct Elektrother Res 2: 237–246
7. Angaut-Petit D (1975a) The dorsal column system: I. Existence of long ascending postsynaptic fibers of the cat's fasciculus gracilis. Exp Brain Res 22: 457–470

8. Angaut-Petit D (1975b) The dorsal column system: II. Functional properties and bulbar relay of the post-synaptic fibers of the cat's fasciculus gracilis. Exp Brain Res 22: 471–493
9. Berlin L, Goodell H, Wolff HG (1958) Studies on pain. Relation of pain perception and central inhibitory effect of noxious stimulation to phenomenon of extinction of pain. Arch Neurol 80: 533–543
10. Besson JM, Chaouch A (1987) Peripheral and spinal mechanisms of nociception. Physiol Rev 67: 67–186
11. Bodnar RJ, Kordower JH, Wallace MM, Tamir H (1981) Stress and morphine analgesia: alterations following p-chlorophenylalanine. Pharmacol. Biochem Behav 14: 645–651
12. Bourgoin S, Oliveras JL, Bruxelle J, Hamon M, Besson JM (1980) Electrical stimulation of the nucleus raphe magnus in the rat: effects on 5-HT metabolism in the spinal cord. Brain Res 194: 377–389
13. Boivie J (1979) An anatomical reinvestigation of the termination of the spinothalamic tract in the monkey. J Comp Neurol 186: 343–370
14. Bouhassira D, Le Bars D, Villanueva L (1987) Heterotopic activation of Aδ and C fibers triggers inhibition of trigeminal and spinal convergent neurones in the rat. J Physiol (Lond) 389: 301–317
15. Buckett WR (1979) Peripheral stimulation in mice induces short-duration analgesia preventable by naloxone. Eur J Pharmacol 58: 169–178
16. Buckett WR (1981) Pharmacological studies on stimulation-produced analgesia in mice. Eur J Pharmacol 69: 281–290
17. Burgess PR, Perl ER (1973) Cutaneous mechanoreceptors and nociceptors. In: Iggo A (eds) Handbook of sensory physiology. Springer, Berlin Heidelberg, pp 29–78
18. Cadden SW, Villanueva L, Chitour D, Le Bars D (1983) Depression of activities of dorsal horn convergent neurones by propriospinal mechanisms triggered by noxious inputs; comparison with diffuse noxious inhibitory controls (DNIC). Brain Res 275: 1–11
19. Calvino B, Le Bars D (1986) The response to viscero-peritoneal nociceptive stimuli is reduced in the experimental arthritic rat. Brain Res 370: 191–195
20. Calvino B, Villanueva L, Le Bars D (1984) The heterotopic effects of visceral pain: behavioural and electrophysiological approaches in the rat. Pain 20: 261–271
21. Calvino B, Crepon-Bernard MO, Le Bars D (1987a) Parallel clinical and behavioural studies of adjuvant-induced arthritis in the rat: possible relationship with "chronic pain". Behav Brain Res 24: 11–29
22. Calvino B, Villanueva L, Le Bars D (1987b) Dorsal horn (convergent) neurones in the intact anaesthetized arthritic rat: I. Segmental excitatory influences. Pain 28: 81–98
23. Calvino B, Villanueva L, Le Bars D (1987c) Dorsal horn (convergent) neurones in the intact anaesthetized arthritic rat. II. Heterotopic inhibitory influences. Pain (In press)
24. Chapman DB, Way LE (1982) Modification of endorphin/enkephalin analgesia and stress-induced analgesia by divalent cations, a cation chelator and an ionophore. Br J Pharmacol 75: 389–396
25. Chesher GB, Chan B (1977) Footshock induced analgesia in mice: its reversal by naloxone and cross tolerance with morphine. Life Sci 21: 1569–1574
26. Chiang CY, Chang CT, Chu HL, Yang LF (1973) Peripheral afferent pathway for acupuncture analgesia. Sci Sin [B] 16: 210–217
27. Chiang CY, Liu JY, Chu TH, Pai YH, Chang SC (1975) Studies on spinal ascending pathway for effect of acupuncture analgesia in rabbits. Sci Sin [B] 18: 651–658
28. Chitour D, Dickenson AH, Le Bars D (1982) Pharmacological evidence for the involvement of serotonergic mechanism in diffuse noxious inhibitory controls (DNIC). Brain Res 236: 329–337
29. Chung JM, Lee KH, Hori Y, Endo K, Willis WD (1984) Factors influencing peripheral nerve stimulation produced inhibition of primate spinothalamic tract cells. Pain 19: 277–293
30. Colpaert FC, Niemegeers CJE, Janssen PAJ (1978) Nociceptive stimulation prevents development of tolerance to narcotic analgesia. Eur J Pharmacol 49: 335–336
31. Colpaert FC, Meert TH, De Witte PH, Schmitt P (1982) Further evidence validating adjuvant arthritis as an experimental model of chronic pain in the rat. Life Sci 31: 67–75
32. Craig Jr AD, Tapper DN (1978) Lateral cervical nucleus in the cat: functional organization and characteristics. J. Neurophysiol 41: 1511–1534

33. Dahlstrom A, Fuxe K (1965) Evidence for the existence of monoamine neuron in the central nervous system: II. Experimentally induced changes in the intraneuronal amine levels of bulbospinal neuron system. Acta Physiol Scand 64 [Suppl] 247: 1-36
34. De Castro Costa M, De Sutter P, Gybels J, Van Hees J (1981) Adjuvant induced arthritis in rats; a possible model of chronic pain. Pain 10: 173-186
35. Department of Physiology, Kirin Medical College, Changchum (1977) The inhibition effect and the mode of action of electroacupuncture upon discharges from the pain-sensitive cells in spinal trigeminal nucleus, Sci Sin [B] 20: 485-501
36. Dickenson AH, Le Bars D (1983) Diffuse noxious inhibitory controls (DNIC) involve trigeminothalamic and spinothalamic neurones in the rat. Exp Brain Res 49: 174-180
37. Dickenson AH, Le Bars D, Besson JM (1980a) Diffuse noxious inhibitory controls (DNIC). Effects on trigeminal nucleus caudalis neurones in the rat. Brain Res 200: 293-305
38. Dickenson AH, Le Bars D, Besson JM (1980b) An involvement of nucleus raphe magnus in diffuse noxious inhibitory controls (DNIC) in the rat. Neurosci Lett [Suppl] 5: 375
39. Dickenson AH, Rivot JP, Chaouch A, Besson JM, Le Bars D (1981) Diffuse noxious inhibitory controls (DNIC) in the rat with or without pCPA pretreatment. Brain Res 216: 313-321
40. Du HJ, Chao YF (1976) Localization of central structures involved in descending inhibitory effects of acupuncture on viscero-somatic discharges. Sci Sin [B] 19: 137-148
41. Dubner R, Beitel E (1976) Peripheral neural correlates of escape behavior in rhesus monkey to noxious heat applied to the face. In: Bonica JJ, Albe-Fessard D (eds) Advances in pain research and therapy, vol 1. Raven, New York, pp 155-160
42. Duchenne GBA (1855) De l'électrisation localisée et de son application à la physiologie, à la pathologie et à la thérapeutique. Baillière, Paris
43. Duncker K (1937) Some preliminary experiments on the mutual influence of pains. Psychologische Forschung 21: 311-326
44. Eriksson M, Sjolund B (1976) Acupuncturelike electroanalgesia in TNS-resistant chronic pain. In: Zotterman Y (eds) Sensory functions of the skin in primates. Pergamon, Oxford, pp 575-582
45. Fitzgerald M (1982) The contralateral input to the dorsal horn of the spinal cord in the decerebrate spinal rat. Brain Res 236: 275-287
46. Foerster O, Gagel O (1931) Die Vorderseitenstrang durch Schneidung beim Menschen. Eine Klinisch-pathophysiologisch-anatomische Studie. Z Ges Neurol Psychiatr 138: 1-92
47. Fox EJ, Melzack R (1976a) Comparison of transcutaneous electrical stimulation and acupuncture in the treatment of chronic pain. In: Bonica JJ, Albe-Fessard D (eds) Advances in pain research and therapy, vol 1. Raven, New York, pp 797-801
48. Fox EJ, Melzack R (1976b) Transcutaneous electrical stimulation and acupuncture: comparison of treatment for low-back pain. Pain 2: 141-148
49. Gammon GD, Starr I (1941) Studies on the relief of pain by counter-irritation. J Clin Invest 20: 13-20
50. Gasser HS, Erlanger J (1927) The role played by the sizes of the constituent fibers of a nerve trunk in determining the form of its action potential wave. Am J Physiol 80: 522-547
51. Gehrart KD, Yezierski RP, Giesler Jr GJ, Willis WD (1981) Inhibitory receptive fields of primate spinothalamic tract cells. J Neurophysiol 46: 1309-1325
52. Giesler Jr GJ, Cliffer KD (1985) Post-synaptic dorsal column pathway of the rat: II. Evidence against an important role in nociception. Brain Res 326: 347-356
53. Giesler Jr GJ, Menétrey D, Basbaum AI (1979) Differential origins of spinothalamic tract projections to medial and lateral thalamus in the rat. J Comp Neurol 184: 107-126
54. Giesler Jr GJ, Spiel HR, Willis WD (1981) Organization of spinothalamic tract axons within the rat spinal cord. J Comp Neurol 195: 243-252
55. Giesler Jr GJ, Nahin RL, Madsen A (1984) Post-synaptic dorsal column pathway of the rat: I. Anatomical studies. J Neurophysiol 51: 260-275
56. Grant AE (1964) Massage with ice (cryokinetics) in the treatment of painful conditions of the musculoskeletal pain. Arch Phys Med Rehabil 45: 233-238
57. Guilbaud G, Iggo A, Tegner R (1985) Sensory receptors in ankle joint capsules of normal and arthritic rats. Exp Brain Res 58: 29-40
58. Gybels J, Handwerker HO, Van Hees J (1979) Comparison between the discharges of human

nociceptive nerve fibres and the subject's rating of his sensation. J Physiol (Lond) 292: 193–206

59. Hammond DL, Tyce GM, Yaksh TL (1985) Efflux of 5-hydroxytryptamine and noradrenaline into spinal cord superfusates during stimulation of the rat medulla. J Physiol (Lond) 359: 151–162

60. Han JS, Terenius L (1982) Neurochemical basis of acupuncture analgesia. Annu Rev Pharmacol Toxicol 22: 193–220

61. Hardy JD, Wolff HG, Goodell H (1940) Studies on pain. A new method for measuring pain threshold: observations on spatial summation of pain. J Clin Invest 19: 649–657

62. Hardy JD, Goodell H, Wolff HG (1951) The influence of skin temperature upon the pain threshold as evoked by thermal radiation. Science 114: 149–150

63. Hayes RL, Bennett GJ, Newlon PG, Mayer DJ (1978) Behavioral and physiological studies of non-narcotic analgesia in the rat elecitied by certain environmental stimuli. Brain Res 155: 69–90

64. Hazouri LA, Mueller AD (1950) Pain threshold studies on paraplegic patients. Arch Neurol Psychiatr 64: 607–613

65. He L (1987) Involvement of endogenous opioid peptides in acupuncture analgesia. Pain 31: 99–121

66. Hutson PH, Tricklebank MD, Curzon G (1982) Enhancement of footshock-induced analgesia by spinal 5,7-dihydroxytryptamine lesions. Brain Res 237: 367–372

67. Jeans ME (1979) Relief of chronic pain by brief, intense transcutaneous electrical stimulation – a double-blind study. In: Bonica JJ, Liebeskind JC, Albe-Fessard (eds) Advances in pain research and therapy, vol 3. Raven, New York, pp 601–606

68. Kane K, Taub A (1975) A history of local electrical analgesia. Pain 1: 125–138

69. Kawakita K, Funakoshi M (1982) Suppression of the jaw-opening reflex by conditioning A-delta fiber stimulation and electroacupuncture in the rat. Exp Neurol 78: 461–465

70. Kerr FWL (1975) The ventral spinothalamic tract and other ascending systems of the ventral funiculus of the spinal cord. J Comp Neurol 159: 335–356

71. Kraus E, Le Bars D, Besson JM (1981) Behavioral confirmation of "diffuse noxious inhibitory controls" (DNIC) and evidence for a role of endogenous opiates. Brain Res 206: 495–499

72. Kraus E, Besson JM, Le Bars D (1982) Behavioural model for diffuse noxious inhibitory controls (DNIC): potentiation by 5-hydroxytryptophan. Brain Res 231: 461–465

73. Kugelberg E (1952) Facial reflexes. Brain 75: 385–396

74. Lagerweij E, Nelis PC, Wiegant VM, Van Ree JM (1984) The twitch in horses: a variant of acupuncture. Science 225: 1172–1174

75. Lamotte RH, Campbell JN (1978) Comparison of responses of warm and nociceptive C fiber afferent in monkey with human judgements of thermal pain. J Neurophysiol 41: 509–528

76. Le Bars D (1988) Serotonin and pain. In: Osborne N, Hamon M (eds) Neuronal Serotonin. Wiley, Chichester (In press)

77. Le Bars D, Dickenson AH, Besson JM (1979a) Diffuse noxious inhibitory controls (DNIC): I. Effects on dorsal horn convergent neurones in the rat. Pain 6: 283–304

78. Le Bars D, Dickenson AH, Besson JM (1979b) Dissue noxious inhibitory controls (DNIC): II. Lack of effect on non convergent neurones, supraspinal involvement and theoretical implications. Pain 6: 305–327

79. Le Bars D, Chitour D, Clot AM (1981a) The encoding of thermal stimuli by diffuse noxious inhibitory controls (DNIC). Brain Res 230: 394–399

80. Le Bars D, Chitour D, Kraus E, Dickenson AH, Besson JM (1981b) Effect of naloxone upon diffuse noxious inhibitory controls (DNIC) in the rat. Brain Res 204: 387–402

81. Le Bars D, Calvino B, Villanueva L, Cadden S (1984) Physiological approaches to counter-irritation phenomena. In: Tricklebank MD, Curzon G (eds) Stress-induced analgesia. Wiley, Chichester, pp 67–101

82. Le Bars D, Dickenson AH, Besson JM, Villanueva L (1986) Aspects of sensory processing through convergent neurons. In: Yaksh TL (ed) Spinal afferent processing. Plenum, New York, pp 467–504

83. Le Bars D, Bourgoin S, Clot AM, Hamon M, Cesselin F (1987a) Noxious mechanical stimuli

109

increase the release of Met-enkephalin-like material heterosegmentally in the rat spinal cord. Brain Res 402: 181-192

84. Le Bars D, Bourgoin S, Villanueva L, Clot AM, Hamon M, Cesselin F (1987b) Involvement of the dorsolateral funiculi in the spinal release of Met-enkephalin-like material triggered by heterosegmental noxious mechanical stimuli. Brain Res 412: 190-195

85. Lee HK, Chung JM, Willis WD (1985) Inhibition of primate spinothalamic tract cells by TENS. J Neeurosurg 2: 276-287

86. Levine JD, Gormley J, Fields HL (1976) Observations on the analgesic effects of needle puncture (acupuncture). Pain 2: 149-159

87. Lewis JW, Cannon JT, Liebeskind JC (1980) Opioid and non-opioid mechanisms of stress analgesia. Science 208: 623-625

88. Lewis JW, Sherman JE, Liebeskind JC (1981) Opioid and non-opioid stress analgesia: assessment of tolerance and cross-tolerance with morphine. J Neurosci 4: 358-363

89. Lipman JJ, Blumenkopf B, Parris WCV (1987) Chronic pain assessment using the heat beam dolorimetry. Pain 30: 59-67

90. Lundberg A, Oscarsson O (1961) Three ascending spinal pathways in the dorsal part of the lateral funiculus. Acta Physiol Scand 51: 1-16

91. Mann F (1974) Acupuncture analgesia, report of 100 experiments. Br J Anaesth 46: 361-364

92. Mehler WR (1969) Some neurological species differences - a posteriori. Ann NY Acad Sci 167: 424-468

93. Mehler WR, Feferman ME, Nauta WJH (1960) Ascending axon degeneration following anterolateral cordotomy: an experimental study in monkey. Brain 83: 718-750

94. Melzack R (1975) Prolonged relief of pain by brief, intense transcutaneous somatic stimulation. Pain 1: 357-373

95. Melzack R (1984) Acupuncture and related forms of folk medicine. In: Wall PD, Melzack R (eds) Textbook of pain. Churchill Livingstone, Edinburgh, pp 691-700

96. Melzack R, Wall PD (1965) Pain mechanisms: a new theory. Science 150: 971-979

97. Melzack R, Stillwell DM, Fox EJ (1977) Trigger points and acupuncture points for pain: correlations and implications. Pain 3: 3-24

98. Melzack R, Guite S, Gonshor A (1980a) Relief of dental pain by ice massage of the hand. Can Med Assoc J 122: 189-191

99. Melzack R, Jeans ME, Stratford JG, Monks RC (1980b) Ice massage and transcutaneous electrical stimulation: comparison of treatment for low-back pain. Pain 9: 209-217

100. Menétrey D, Besson JM (1982) Electrophysiological characteristics of dorsal horn cells in rats with cutaneous inflammation resulting from chronic arthritis. Pain 13: 343-364

101. Mennell JM (1975) The therapeutic use of cold. J Am Osteopath Assoc 74: 1146-1158

102. Merskey H, Evans PR (1975) Variations in pain complaint threshold in psychiatric and neurological patients with pain. Pain 1: 73-79

103. Morin F (1955) A new spinal pathway for cutaneous impulses. Am J Physiol 183: 245-252

104. Morton CR, Maisch B, Zimmerman M (1987) Diffuse noxious inhibitory controls of lumbar spinal neurons involve a supraspinal loop in the cat. Brain Res 410: 347-352

105. Nathan PW, Rudge P (1974) Testing the gate-control theory of pain in man. J Neurol Neurosurg Psychiatry 37: 1366-1372

106. Noordenbos W (1959) Pain, Elsevier, Amsterdam

107. Parsons CM, Goetzl FR (1945) Effect of induced pain on pain threshold. Proc Soc Exp Biol Med 60: 327-329

108. Pertovaara A, Kemppainen P, Johansson G, Karonen SL (1982) Ischemic pain nonsegmentally produces a predominant reduction of pain and thermal sensitivity in man: a selective role for endogenous opioids. Brain Res 251: 83-92

109. Peschanski M, Guilbaud G, Lam Lee C, Mantyh PW (1983) Involvement of the rat ventrobasal thalamic complex in the sensory-discriminative aspect of pain: electrophysiological and anatomical data. In: Macchi G, Rustioni A, Spreafico R (eds) Somatosensory integration in the thalamus. Elsevier, Amsterdam pp 147-163

110. Pilowsky PM, Kapoor V, Minson JB, West MJ, Chalmers JP (1986) Spinal cord serotonin release and raised blood pressure after brainstem kainic acid injection. Brain Res 366: 354-357

110

111. Pircio A, Fedele CT, Bierwagen ME (1975) A new method for the evaluation of analgesic activity using adjuvant induced arthritis in the rat. Eur J Pharmacol 31: 207–215

112. Rivot JP, Chaouch A, Besson JM (1979) The influence of naloxone on the C-fiber response of dorsal horn neurons and their inhibitory control by raphe magnus stimulation. Brain Res 176: 355–364

113. Rivot JP, Chiang CY, Besson JM (1982) Increase in serotonin metabolism within the dorsal horn of the spinal cord during nucleus raphe magnus stimulation, as revealed by in vivo electrochemical detection. Brain Res 238: 1117–1126

114. Roby-Brami A, Bussel B, Willer JC, Le Bars D (1987) An electrophysiological investigation into the pain-relieving effects of heterotopic nociceptive stimuli: possible involvement of a supraspinal loop. Brain 110: 69–80

115. Sarlandiére JB (1825) Mémoires sur l'electro-puncture. Paris

116. Satran R, Goldstein MN (1973) Pain perception: modification of threshold of intolerance and cortical potentials by cutaneous stimulation. Science 180: 1201–1202

117. Shangai Acupuncture Anesthesia Co-ordinating Group (1977) Acupuncture anesthesia: an anesthetic method combining traditional Chinese and Western medicine. Comp Med East West 5: 301–313

118. Shen E, Tsai TT, Lan C (1975) Supraspinal participation in the inhibitory effect of acupuncture on viscero-somatic reflex discharges. Chin Med J [Engl] 1: 431–440

119. Schouenborg J, Dickenson A (1985) The effects of a distant noxious stimulation on A and C fiber evoked flexion reflexes and neuronal activity in dorsal horn of the rat. Brain Res 328: 23–32

120. Sjolund BH (1985) Peripheral nerve suppression of C-fiber-evoked flexion reflex in rats. Part I: parameters of continuous stimulation. J Neurosurg 63: 612–616

121. Skagerberg G, Bjorklund A (1985) Topographic principles in the spinal projections of serotonergic and non-serotonergic brainstem neurons in the rat. Neuroscience 15: 445–480

122. Talbot JD, Duncan GH, Bushnell MC, Boyer M (1987) Diffuse noxious inhibitory controls (DNICs): psychophysical evidence in man for intersegmental suppression of noxious heat perception by cold pressor pain. Pain 30: 221–232

123. Torebjork H.E., Lamotte RH, Robinson C (1984) Peripheral neural correlates of magnitude of cutaneous pain and hyperalgesia: simultaneous recordings in humans of sensory judgements of pain and evoked responses in nociceptors with C-fibers. J Neurophysiol 51: 325–329

124. Travell J, Rinzler SH (1952) The myofascial genesis of pain. Postgrad Medicine 11: 425–434

125. Tricklebank MD, Hutson PH, Curzon G (1982) Analgesia induced by brief foot-shock is inhibited by 5-hydroxytryptamine but unaffected by antagonists of 5-hydroxytryptamine or naloxone. Neuropharmacology 21: 51–56

126. Trousseau A, Pidoux H (1836–1839) Electricité. Acupuncture. Electroacupuncture. In: Traité de Thérapeutique et de Matiére Medicale vol 1. Bechet Jeune, Paris, pp 742–823

127. Tyce GM, Yaksh TL (1981) Monoamine release from cat spinal cord by somatic stimuli: an intrinsic modulatory system. J Physiol (Lond) 314: 513–529

128. Uddenberg N (1968) Functional organization of long, second-order afferents in the dorsal funiculus. Exp Brain Res 4: 377–382

129. Van Hees J, Gybels JM (1972) Pain related to single afferent C fibers from human skin. Brain Res 48: 397–400

130. Van Hees J, Gybels J (1981) C-nociceptor activity in human nerve during painful and non painful skin stimulation. J Neurol Neurosurg Psychiatry 44: 600–607

131. Villanueva L, Le Bars D (1985) The encoding of thermal stimuli applied to the tail of the rat by lowering the excitability of trigeminal convergent neurones. Brain Res 330: 245–251

132. Villanueva L, Cadden SW, Le Bars D (1984a) Evidence that diffuse noxious inhibitory controls (DNIC) are mediated by a final post-synaptic inhibitory mechanism. Brain Res 298: 67–74

133. Villanueva L, Cadden SW, Le Bars D (1984b) Diffuse noxious inhibitory controls (DNIC): evidence for post-synaptic inhibition of trigeminal nucleus caudalis convergent neurones. Brain Res 321: 165–168

134. Villanueva L, Peschanski M, Calvino B, Le Bars D (1986a) Ascending pathways in the spinal

111

cord involved in triggering of diffuse noxious inhibitory controls (DNIC) in the rat. J Neurophysiol 55: 34–55

135. Villanueva L, Chitour D, Le Bars D (1986b) Involvement of the dorsolateral funiculus in the descending spinal projections responsible for diffuse noxious inhibitory controls in the rat. J Neurophysiol 56: 1185–1195
136. Wall PD, Sweet WH (1967) Temporary abolition of pain in man. Science 155: 108–109
137. Wand-Tetley JI (1956) Historical methods of counter-irritation. Ann Phys Med 3: 90–98
138. Watkins LR, Cobelli DA, Faris P, Aceto MD, Mayer DJ (1982) Opiate vs non-opiate footshock-induced analgesia (FSIA): the body region shocked is a critical factor. Brain Res 242: 299–308
139. Watkins LR, Mayer DJ (1982) Involvement of spinal opioid systems in footshock-induced analgesia: antagonism by naloxone is possible only before induction of analgesia. Brain Res 242: 309–316
140. Weil-Fugazza J, Godefroy F, Le Bars D (1984) Increase in 5-HT synthesis in the dorsal part of the spinal cord, induced by a nociceptive stimulus: blockade by morphine. Brain Res 297: 247–264
141. Willer JC (1977) Comparative study of perceived pain and nociceptive flexion reflex in man. Pain 3: 69–80
142. Willer JC, Lamour Y (1975) analyse électrophysiologique du réflexe de clignement chèz le singe. CR Acad Sci [III] 281: 563–566
143. Willer JC, Boureau F, Albe-Fessard D (1978) Role of large diameter cutaneous afferents in transmission of nociceptive messages: electrophysiological study in man. Brain Res 152: 358–364
144. Willer JC, Roby A, Boulu P, Boureau F (1982a) Comparative effects of electroacupuncture and transcutaneous stimulation on the human blink reflex. Pain 14: 267–278
145. Willer JC, Roby A, Boulu P, Albe-Fessard D (1982b) Depressive effect of high frequency peripheral conditioning stimulation upon the nociceptive component of the human blink reflex. Lack of naloxone effect. Brain Res 239: 322–326
146. Willer JC, Roby A, Le Bars D (1984) Psychophysical and electrophysiological approaches to the pain relieving effect of heterotopic nociceptive stimuli. Brain 107: 1095–1112
147. Willer JC, Barranquero A, Kahn MF, Sallière D (1987) Pain in sciatica depresses lower limb cutaneous reflexes to sural nerve stimulation. J Neurol Neurosurg Psychiatry 50:1–5
148. Willis WD, Kenshalo Jr DR, Leonard RB (1979) The cells of origin of the primate spinothalamic tract. J Comp Neurol 188: 543–574
149. Woolf CJ, Mitchell D, Barrett GD (1980) Antinociceptive effect of peripheral segmental electrical stimulation in the rat. Pain 8: 237–252
150. Zemlan FD, Leonard CM, Kow LM, Pfaff DW (1978) Ascending tracts of the lateral columns of the rat spinal cord: a study using the silver impregnation and horseradish peroxidase techniques. Exp Neurol 62: 298–334

Activation of the Enkephalinergic System by Acupuncture

Kang Tsou

Shanghai Institute of Materia Medica, Chinese Academy of Sciences, Shanghai 200031, People's Republic of China

Ever since the discovery of enkephalins by Hughes, Kosterlitz, et al. [1], several laboratories in China have been working on the involvement of endogenous opioid peptides in acupuncture analgesia, notably Han's group in Beijing [2] and Zhang's group [3] in Shanghai. My laboratory first studied 5-hydroxytryptamine (5-HT) involvement in acupuncture analgesia, and then attention was focussed on the role of enkephalins.

The role of 5-Hydroxytryptamine in Acupuncture Analgesia

The acupuncture analgesia project was started in 1973 with the role of 5-HT. Morphine was always used as an experimental control. Using rabbit as the experimental model, the release of 5-HT during acupuncture was studied [4]. Pain sensitivity was measured by potassium ionophoresis on the ear tips through two cotton wick electrodes, one on each ear. The current passing through the ears was increased steadily, and the current that caused a sudden struggle of the rabbit was recorded as the pain threshold. Plastic cannulas were implanted in the rabbits, one in the lateral ventricle and another in the aqueduct. The rabbits were suspended in cloth slings. The ventricular system was perfused with [^{3}H]5-HT-containing artificial CSF, during which time [^{3}H]5-HT was presumably taken up by the serotonergic nerve endings. The perfusion was then continued with [^{3}H]5-HT-free CSF. Under control conditions, the radioactivity in the perfusates (collected at 10-min intervals) decreased in a time-dependent fashion. If the rabbits were manually acupunctured by twirling needles in the St.36 Zusanli points of both hind legs for 20 min, the radioactivity in the perfusates increased concomitantly with the elevation of the pain threshold. Iv injection of morphine (5 mg/kg), by contrast, produced a prominent and long-lasting elevation of the pain threshold without any increase of radioactivity in the perfusates. Therefore, there is a distinct difference between acupuncture and morphine analgesia with regard to 5-HT.

The effect of chemical lesioning of serotonergic neurons on acupuncture analgesia was also studied [5]. The 5-HT neurotoxin 5,6-dihydroxytryptamine (5,6-DHT) was first injected into the lateral ventricle of the rat 1 week prior to assessment of the analgesic effect of electroacupuncture. The pain threshold was measured using the tail-flick test. Electroacupuncture was induced by application of high- and low-frequency impulses through needle electrodes inserted in the Gb.30 Huantiao points on both hind legs. This procedure caused a conspicuous increase in the tail-flick latency in control rats. The analgesia of electroacupuncture was significantly attenuated in 5,6-DHT-treated rats. Histochemical examination of the raphe nucleus in these rats revealed degeneration of the cell bodies, swelling of axons, and loss of fluorescence in the nerve terminals.

The Role of Opioid Peptides in Acupuncture Analgesia

After the important discovery of enkephalins, I started working on the role of enkephalins in acupuncture analgesia. I was further encouraged by the work of Mayer et al. [4] that naloxone could partially antagonize acupuncture analgesia and the paper by Sjolund et al. [5] that electroacupuncture increased the level of endogenous opioids in the lumbar CSF in patients. Since either naloxone or radio-receptor binding assay was used in these two papers, it was not possible to identify which opioid peptide(s) was involved. Therefore, a radioimmunoassay was developed for Leu- and Met-enkephalin [8]. The immunogens were prepared by condensation of polylysyl succinic acid with the N-terminals of the two enkephalins. My Leu-enkephalin antiserum could detect 20 pg Leu-enkephalin, while the Met-enkephalin antiserum could detect 150 pg Met-enkephalin.

Alteration of Brain Regional Enkephalin Contents by Acupuncture

Using these antisera, the regional contents of Leu- and Met-enkephalins were measured before and after acupuncture [9]. In the rabbit experiments, after alternately twirling acupuncture needles in the bilateral St.36 Zusanli points for 20 min, the pain threshold usually increased more than 80% as measured by potassium ionophoresis on the rabbit ear. The rabbit was then decapitated and the brain dissected into the following regions: hypothalamus, striatum, hippocampus, thalamus, brain stem, and cortex. The enkephalin contents were measured by radioimmunoassay with these antisera. In the control group, enkephalin contents were high in the hypothalamus and the striatum. After acupuncture, there were prominent increases in these two regions of about 1.6–1.8-fold. No significant changes were found in other regions. In the rat experiments, the pain threshold as measured 5 s after 30 min of electroacupuncture increased 92%. Most prominent changes in enkephalin levels were again found in the hypothalamus and the striatum. Compared with the control group, Met-enkephalin increased 3.5 times, while Leu-enkephalin increased 1.4–2 times.

Immunohistochemical data obtained independently by Watson et al. [10] and Bloom et al. [11] showed that the β-endorphin neuronal system is located separately from the enkephalin neurons. The β-endorphin cells are located mainly in the basal hypothalamus. The Halasz knife was therefore used to isolate the basal hypothalamus from the rest of the brain. The effect of such an isolation on acupuncture analgesia and the Met-enkephalin content in the basal hypothalamus was studied. Thirty rats were divided into the following groups: (a) control, (b) hypothalamus isolation, (c) hypothalamus isolation plus electroacupuncture, (d) sham operation, and (e) sham operation plus electroacupuncture. Rats in group e showed a prominent increase of the pain threshold. Rats in group c showed less effective analgesia. The Met-enkephalin content in the isolated hypothalamus was about the same in the hypothalamus of sham-operated rats, but electroacupuncture failed to increase the Met-enkephalin content in the isolated hypothalamus, indicating that the incoming impulses were essential for the acupuncture-induced enkephalin elevation [12].

Effect of the Peptidase Inhibitor Bacitracin on Acupuncture Analgesia

It is well-known that acupuncture only produces a transient analgesia in animals and that enkephalins degrade rapidly after release. If enkephalins are indeed involved in acupuncture analgesia, delaying their degradation should prolong the analgesia. Therefore I injected the peptidase inhibitor bacitracin 50 μg/50 μl into the lateral ventricle of the rabbit and found that the acupuncture analgesia was conspicuously prolonged. The elevated pain threshold of rabbits injected with saline returned to the preacupuncture level 30–40 min after the cessation of acupuncture, while the pain threshold in the bacitracin plus acupuncture group was still markedly elevated [13]. When the rabbits were killed 30–40 min after the cessation of acupuncture, the enkephalin contents in the hypothalamus and the striatum were found to be highest in the bacitracin plus acupuncture group and lowest in the bacitracin control. The saline plus acupuncture group showed a residual elevation. These results indicate that the enkephalinergic neurons have a low level of activity during the resting state. Iv administered naloxone was capable of reversing the acupuncture analgesia during the bacitracin-prolonged analgesia period, implying that the prolongation is due to endogenous opioid substances.

Release of Brain Enkephalins by Acupuncture

To discover whether acupuncture releases brain enkephalins, the Met-enkephalin content in the rabbit CSF was measured [14]. Experiments were performed in bacitracin alone and bacitracin plus acupuncture groups. The pain threshold was still highly elevated in the latter group 30 min after the cessation of acupuncture. Cisternal CSF was sampled at this time, and the Met-enkephalin content was found to be significantly higher in the bacitracin plus acupuncture group, indicating that acupuncture activated the enkephalinergic neurons to release enkephalin into the CSF. Likewise, a similar increase of Met-enkephalin content in the CSF of the monkeys was found after electroacupuncture [15].

Dynamic Changes in the Release and Biosynthesis of Enkephalins After Acupuncture

It was reported that the protein synthesis inhibitor cycloheximide interfered with the incorporation of tritium-labelled tyrosine into enkephalins in vitro [16]. I studied its in vivo effect on acupuncture analgesia after intraventricular injection. The dose of cycloheximide was 500 pg per rat. This drug alone had no discernible effect on the pain threshold but greatly attenuated the electroacupuncture analgesia. It also decreased the Met-enkephalin content by 47% in the hypothalamus and by 20% in the striatum. In the electroacupuncture group, the Met-enkephalin level increased 113% in the hypothalamus and 200% in the striatum, but in the cycloheximide plus acupuncture group, it increased only 28% and 120%, respectively. The amplitude of the Met-enkephalin increase by acupuncture was greatly reduced by cycloheximide, suggesting that acupuncture accelerates enkephalin biosynthesis [17].

To study further the dynamic changes in the biosynthesis and release of enkephalins in acupuncture, high-potassium-induced enkephalin release from the in vitro striatal slices of control and electroacupuncture-treated rats was studied [18]. Rats were decapitated immediately, 15, 30, or 60 min after the termination of 30-min electric acupuncture treatment. Striatal slices 150–200 μm thick and weighing 30 mg were perfused with Krebs solution in a perfusing chamber. Perfusates collected at 2-min intervals were used for Leu-enkephalin radioimmunoassay. When the striatal slices from control rats were perfused with a Krebs solution containing 30 mM potassium, Leu-enkephalin release was observed after a 2-min delay, attaining its peak rate in 3 min, decreasing gradually thereafter, and approaching the basal rate in 7 min. In the group of rats killed immediately after the termination of the 30-min electroacupuncture treatment, the striatal slices became refractory to high potassium stimulation. There was a partial recovery of potassium-induced Leu-enkephalin release in the group of rats killed 15 min after the cessation of treatment. A full recovery was seen in the 60-min group. In view of the fact that the enkephalin content was actually increased in the rats killed immediately, the demonstration of decreased potassium-induced Leu-enkephalin release was rather surprising. However, it might be explained if the possibility of enkephalin having two pools, is considered, one releasable and the other nonreleasable. A long period of electroacupuncture depletes the releasable pool, while accelerating the biosynthesis and the processing of the enkephalin precursors. The newly formed enkephalin would take 30–60 min to become releasable.

To substantiate this working hypothesis that acupuncture accelerates enkephalin biosynthesis, the level of high molecular weight enkephalin-containing precursors were directly measured after electroacupuncture treatment [19]. Leu-enkephalin and its precursors in the pooled striatal extracts of 10 rats were first fractionated on a Sephadex G-75 column according to Lewis et al. [20]. The eluates were collected at 2-min intervals. Two peaks representing large and small molecular weight peptides were monitored by absorbance at 254 nm. The first peak was in the void volume while the second peak was in the salt volume. Leu-enkephalin could be detected directly in the eluates corresponding to the second peak. The immunoreactivity in the first peak and the intermediate region was detected only after trypsin and carboxypeptidase B digestion. Leu-enkephalin immunoreactrivities in the first peak, the intermediate region, and the second peak were counted as the enkephalin precursor, the processed intermediates, and the free Leu-enkephalin, respectively. Their levels were measured in the following groups, each containing 10 rats: control, killed immediately, 0.25, 0.5, 1, 2, 4, 8, 16, 24, 48, 96 h after the termination of 30-min electroacupuncture. The Leu-enkephalin level was very markedly elevated in the 0-h group, decreased gradually in the 0.25-, 0.5- and 1-h groups. In the 2- and 4-h groups, the Leu-enkephalin level was below that of the control group. From 8 h onward, the Leu-enkephalin level again increased steadily but was never as high as in the 0-h group. The proenkephalin and intermediates levels showed no change in the 0-, 0.25-, and 0.5-h groups but started to increase after 1 h. Their levels became steadily higher until 96 h. This increase in the proenkephalin and intermediates levels preceded the second phase of Leu-enkephalin elevation.

Hybridization Approaches to Study the Role of Enkephalins in Acupuncture Analgesia

In order to learn whether or not acupuncture acceleration of enkephalin biosynthesis also involves the transcriptional level, the proenkephalin mRNA quantity in the rat striatum was measured by the recombinant DNA technique [21]. The proenkephalin mRNA was hybridized by a dot-blot procedure with a 918-base pair cDNA sequence complementary to human pheochromocytoma proenkephalin mRNA kindly donated by Prof. E.Herbert. Rats receiving electroacupuncture treatment showed a three- to fivefold increase of proenkephalin mRNA in the striatum, beginning 1 h after the cessation of the 30-min treatment period and lasting for at least 48 h. A threefold increase of proenkephalin mRNA in the pituitary was found immediately after treatment and a five- to sixfold increase at 1 or 24 h after treatment termination. A similar change in adrenal proenkephalin mRNA was also seen after electroacupuncture treatment.

For comparison, the proopiomelanocortin mRNA level in the pituitary and the hypothalamus was also measured by dot-blot hybridization with a ME 150 plasmid containing a 144-base pair cDNA sequence complementary to the lipotropin-coding portion of mouse proopiomelanocortin mRNA (a gift from Prof. E. Herbert). A 50% increase in the proopiomelanocortin mRNA level in the pituitary was observed 1 h after the cessation of the 30-min electroacupuncture treatment. This elevation continued for 96 h with a maximum of about 70% increase at 24 h [22].

Summary and Conclusion

Enkephalins are likely to play an important role in mediating acupuncture analgesia. Acupuncture has proven to be a powerful method to activate the enkephalinergic system. The biosynthesis and posttranslational processing of the enkephalin precursors are accelerated by acupuncture. This activation also involves the transcriptional level as shown by the increase in the proenkephalin mRNA levels in the brain, the pituitary, and the adrenal gland.

References

1. Hughes J, Smith TW, Kosterlitz HW, Fothergill LA, Morgan BA, Morris HR (1975) Identification of two related pentapeptides from brain with potent opiate antagonist activity. Nature 258: 577
2. Han JS (1984) Progress in the pharmacological studies of acupuncture analgesia. Luphar 9th International Congress of Pharmacology Proceedings, London, 1: 287
3. Zhang AZ, Xu SF, Pan XP, Chen JS, Mo WY (1980) Endorphins and acupuncture analgesia. Chin Med J [Engl] 34: 673
4. Mayer DJ, Price DD, Rafii A (1977) Antagonism of acupuncture analgesia in man by the narcotic antagonist naloxone. Brain Res 121: 368
5. Sjolund B, Eriksson M (1977) Increased CSR levels of endorphins after acupuncture. Acta Physiol Scand 100: 382
6. Yi CC, Lu TH, Wu SH, Tsou K (Zou G) (1977) A study on the release of [^{3}H]5-hydroxytryptamine from brain during acupuncture and morphine analgesia. Sci Sin [B] 20: 113
7. Yi CC, Wu SH, Yu YK, Wang FS, Ji XQ, Zhao DD, Tsou K, Zou G (1977) Effect on acupuncture analgesia by intraventricular injection of 5,6-dihydroxtryptamine. A functional and fluorescence histochemical study. Kexue Tongbao 22: 43
8. Lo ES, Wu JB, Yi CC, Wang FS, Zou G (1980) Radioimmunoassay for enkephalins. Acta Biochim Biophys Sin 12: 115
9. Tsou KK (Zou G), Yi CC, Wang FS, Lo ES, Zhang ZX, Wu SX (1980) Alterations of enkephalin contents in brain areas by acupuncture. Kexue Tongbao 25: 78
10. Watson SJ, Akil H, Richard CN, Barchas JD (1978) Evidence for two separate opiate peptide neuronal systems and the coexistence of beta-lipotropin, beta-endorphin and ACTH immunoreactivities in the same hypothalamus neurons. Nature 275: 226
11. Bloom FE, Battenberg E, Rossier J, Ling N, Guillemin R (1978) Neurons containing beta-endorphin in rat brain exist separately from those containing enkephalins. Immunocytochemical studies. Proc Natl Acad Sci USA 75: 1591
12. Tsou K (Zou G), Yi CC, Wu SX, Wang FS, Lo ES, Ji XQ, Yu YK, Zhao DD (1980) Enkephalin involvement in acupuncture analgesia-radioimmunoassay. Sci Sin [B] 23: 1197
13. Tsou K (Zou G), Zhao DD, Wu SX, Zhang ZX, Lo ES, Wang FS (1979) Enhancement of acupuncture analgesia which concomitant increase of enkephalins in striatum and hypothalamus by intraventricular bacitracin. Acta Physiol Sin 31: 377
14. Tsou K (Zou G), Wu SX, Wang FS, Ji XQ, Zhang ZX, Lo ES, Yi CC (1979) Increased levels of endorphins in the cisternal CSF of rabbits in acupuncture analgesia. Acta Physiol Sin 31: 371
15. Huang Y, Xie GY, Wang QW, Wang FS, Tsou K (Zou G) (1982) Increase of enkephalin content in the monkey CSF after electroacupuncture. Kexue Tongbao 27: 449
16. Hughes J, Kosterlitz HW, McKnight AT (1978) The incorporation of [^{3}H]-tyrosine into enkephalin of striatal slices of guinea pig brain. Br J Pharmacol 65: 396
17. Wu SX, Zhang ZX, Wang FS, Tsou K (Zou G) (1980) Effects of intraventricular cycloheximide on acupuncture analgesia and brain Met-enkephalin. Acta Physiol Sin 32: 79
18. Zhu XZ, Wang FS, Yi CC, Tsou K (Zou G) (1985) Decreased potassium induced Leu-enkephalin release from striatal slices after electric acupuncture. Chin J Physiol Sci 1: 146
19. Ding XH, Ji XQ, Tsou K (Zou G) (1986) Dynamic changes in the levels of enkephalin precursors, processed intermediates and Leu-enkephalin in rat caudate nucleus following electroacupuncture. Chin J Physiol Sci 2: 42
20. Lewis RV, Stein S, Gerber LD, Rubinstein M, Udenfriend S (1978) High molecular weight opioid-containing proteins in striatum. Proc Natl Acad Sci USA 75: 4021
21. Zheng M, Yang SL, Tsou K (Zou G) (1987) Electroacupuncture markedly increases proenkephalin mRNA in rat striatum and pituitary. Sci Sin [B] 31: 81
22. Zheng M, Wang LJ, Yang SL, Tsou K (Zou G) (1987) Electroacupuncture increases proopiomelanocortin mRNA in the pituitary and the proenkephalin mRNA in the adrenal gland in the rat. Chin J Physiol Sci 3: 106

Neurophysiology of Electroacupuncture Analgesia

Richard S. S. Cheng

Pain Clinic St. Josephs Hospital and Bathurst Pain Clinic, 800 Bathurst Street, Toronto, Canada

In recent years, electroacupuncture (EA) analgesia has been the focus of intense multidisciplinary research. This research has been very productive, leading to the publication of numerous studies that have added to our understanding of the neurophysiology of pain perception and pain modulation. This article will review the results of some of these studies, from which the central roles in pain modulation played by the endorphins and various monoamines (serotonin, in particular) will become apparent. In conclusion, an integrated neurophysiological model of EA analgesia will be proposed.

Experimental Data Supporting the Acupuncture-Endorphin Hypothesis

Much experimental data support the hypothesis that the analgesia produced by EA is mediated by the release of endorphins into the central nervous system (CNS) and that this release may occur at several different levels within the CNS.

1. An early experiment (Cheng and Pomeranz 1976) involved recording the electrical activity of a single interneuron in lamina V (Rexed) of the spinal cord of an anesthetized cat subjected to peripheral noxious stimulation (i.e., Pinprick). Before discussing the experimental proper, however, it may be useful first to review briefly the functional neuroanatomy. Lamina V of the spinal cord is rich in large interneurons which respond to activity of all three of the main fiber components of the cutaneous nerves: $A\beta$, $A\gamma$, and C fibers. Thus, they respond to both nonnoxious and noxious stimuli and are hence called "wide dynamic range nociceptors." When stimulated by an appropriate noxious stimulus (such as pinpricking the skin, as in the experiment about to be considered), these cells activate ascending dorsal horn nociceptive neurons; the electrical recording of the activity of these interneurons in response to a painful stimulus can therefore be taken as an approximation of the activity of painful signals being sent up to higher brain centers.

Returning now to the EA experiment at hand, electrical recordings were made from such an interneuron in lamina V of the cat's spinal cord under various conditions: subjected to light mechanical stimulation or to noxious pinpricking over the receptive field of the interneuron, both with and without simultaneous application of EA to the same receptive field.

The results are presented in Fig. 1, which shows that: (a) the activity of the interneuron in response to a nonnoxious stimulus was unchanged by EA; and

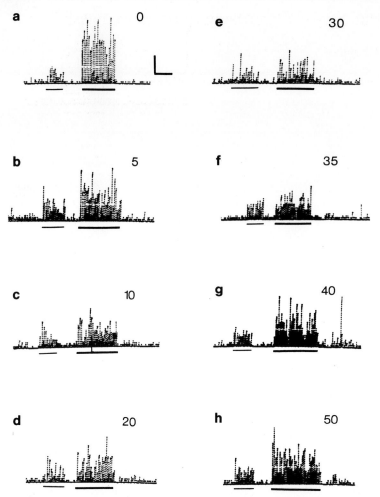

Fig. 1. Records (A to H) from a typical single interneuron in layer 5 of cat spinal cord. The output of an epochal rate meter, bin width 100 msec. is displayed on a storage oscilloscope, each dot representing a single action potential of this cell. As the oscilloscope sweeps from left to right the rate meter produces vertical dots in successively higher positions within bins of 100 msec. A-control before acupuncture; B to E are 5, 10, 20, 30 minutes after onset of acupuncture. F, G and H are recovery taken 35, 40 and 50 minutes; needles are removed at 30 minutes. Horizontal bars indicate the duration of the repetitive stimuli: Thin line is light mechanical stimulus, thick line is noxious pinprick. Scale is 5 sec. horizontal, 50 spikes/sec. vertical

(b) the interneuron's activity in response to noxious stimulation was considerably reduced by continuous EA.

EA-produced inhibition which builds up slowly over time (i.e., EA has a long induction time) and reaches a peak at 30 min; if EA is then discontinued, inhibition of the interneuron is maintained for a considerable length of time, indicating that EA has a prolonged after effect.

Finally, and most importantly, it was also shown (Fig. 2) that the inhibitory

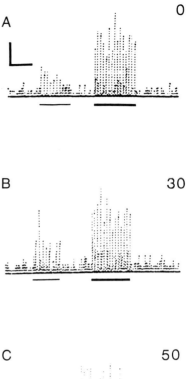

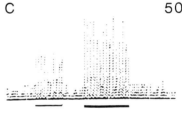

Fig. 2. Records (A to C) from a typical single interneuron in layer 5 of cat spinal cord. The ouput of an epochal rate meter, bin width 100 msec. displayed on a storage oscilloscope, each dot representing a single action potential of this cell. As the oscilloscope sweeps from left to right the rate meter produces vertical dots in successively higher positions within bins of 100 msec. *A* – control before acupuncture and injection of naloxone. *C* – recovery taken 20 min. after needles are removed (Note: electroacupuncture alone was first tested to have a reduction-effect on the noxious response of this typical cell.) *B* – 30 minutes after initiation of acupuncture and injection of naloxone

effect of EA could be blocked by parenteral administration of naloxone (0.3 mg/ kg), which is a potent, almost purely opioid antagonist [24].

Taken together, these results suggest that EA has an inhibitory effect on spinal cord interneurons, that this effect is specific to activity related to the transmission of noxious signals, and that the inhibition may be mediated by opiatelike substances (i.e., endorphins).

2. Microinjections of naloxone (10 µl) into areas of the CNS known to contain endorphins, such as the periaqueductal gray matter (PAG), the caudate nucleus, the nucleus accumbens, or the hypothalamus, all decreased acupuncture analgesia

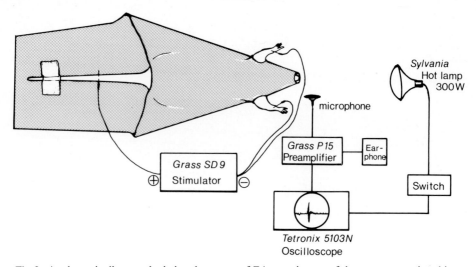

Fig. 3. A schematic diagram depicting the set-up of EA experiments of the mouse restrainted in a paper recepticle. The forelimbs and the tail were immobilized by masking tape. The nose was also exposed to a radiant heat lamp at a distance of 9 cm. Squeak audiogram was recorded by a oscilloscope through a small microphone. Electrical currents were supplied by a Grass SD 9 stimulator. The negative pole was connected to the acupuncture needles inserted into the first dorsal interosseous muscles and positive pole was connected to the needle that was inserted through the middle of the tail

in rats and rabbits, while similar injections into other areas not containing endorphins had no effect [25]. This again suggests that acupuncture produces analgesia via activation of anatomically discrete, opiate-mediated, pain-relieving system that involve many levels of the CNS.

Another series of experiments [4] involving opiate antagonists also were revealing, and these experiments will now be reviewed in some detail.

In this study, the effects of various opiate antagonists on EA analgesia were investigated. EA-treated mice were injected with these various opiate antagonists, and their squeak responses to noxious heat stimulation were recorded; a shortening of the squeak latency period was taken as evidence that the given test substance inhibited EA analgesia. (Refer to Fig. 3 for the experimental set-up.) The animals used for these experiments were B6AF1/J female mice, selected for their reliable squeak response to noxious heat stimulation. The acupuncture needles were placed into the first dorsal interosseous muscles – a placement site required for good EA analgesia.

The experimental results (Figs. 4, 5, 6, 7) suggest that EA is mediated by stereospecific opiate receptors: The type 1 opiate antagonists (i.e., the almost purely opioid antagonists) L-naloxone, naltrexone, and cyclazocine all blocked EA analgesia in these mice, while ther stereoisomer D-naloxone had no effect. These results are further evidence for a specific EA-endorphin relationship.

Using the same experimental set-up (Fig. 3), other studies were performed (Cheng and Pomeranz 1980) to examine the relationship between the frequency of EA and blockage of its analgesia by simultaneous administration of various

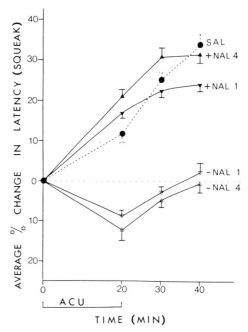

Fig. 4. Effect of (+) naloxone, (−) naloxone or saline on electroacupuncture analgesia in mice. Ordinate shows percentage change in latency to squeak as compared to zero time pretreatment control value. Positive values denote analgesia. + Nal 1 shows effect of electroacupuncture plus dextronaloxone (1 mg/kg). + Nal 4 shows EA plus dextronaloxone (4 mg/kg). Sal shows EA plus saline (0.9%). − Nal 1 shows levonaloxone (1 mg/kg) plus EA. − Nal 4 shows levonaloxone (4 mg/kg) plus EA. Each point is the mean for 15 mice. Bars show standard error. Arrows and 'ACU' indicate time or treatment: EA started after zero time and stopped at 20 minutes; injections were given at zero time and again at 20 minutes (booster). (−) naloxone blocks electroacupuncture analgesia, while saline (0.9%) and (+) naloxone do not

chemicals. It was found (Figs. 8–11) that low-frequency EA (4 Hz) induced an analgesia which could be blocked by naloxone, but that high-frequency EA (200 Hz) induced an analgesia which was not affected by this opiate antagonist. However, it was possible to block partially the high-frequency-induced EA analgesia which injections of parachlorophenylalanine (PCPA), which is an inhibitor of serotonin synthesis. The finding hinted at the existence of another system mediating EA analgesia, to be discussed shortly.

3. Peets and Pomeranz [22] demonstrated that mice (CXBK) genetically deficient in opiate receptors showed poor acupuncture-induced analgesia. They speculated that there are genetic variations in both humans and animals and that because of these a certain proportion (about 30%–40%) of any species will respond poorly to acupuncture due to a poor endorphin system. Support for this idea came when Takeshige [30] observed that those rats (40% of their cohort) demonstrating poor acupuncture analgesia had a deficiency in total brain endorphins, as measured by receptor binding assay.

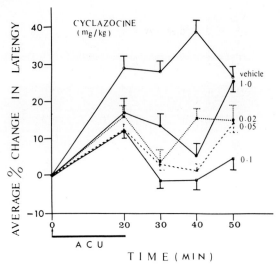

Fig. 5. Effect of cyclazocine on EAA in mice. This diagram is similar to figure 4 except that cyclazocine is administered once (immediately before EA). Doses of cyclazocine for each group of mice are indicated by the numerals 1, 0.1, 0.05 and 0.02 in mg/kg. Each curve represents the mean of 15 mice. Vehicle (0.5 ml/mouse, I. P.) is made by mixing 0.2 ml of 1 N hydrochloric acid and 0.2 ml of 1 N NaOH and the solution is brought to 10 ml with distilled water

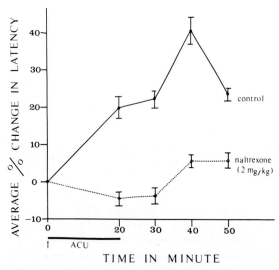

Fig. 6. Effect of naltrexone (2 mg/kg) on EAA in mice. This diagram is similar to Fig. 4 and 5 except naltrexone or 0.9% saline (control) is administered once (immediately before EA indicated by the arrow). Naltrexone reverses EAA in mice

124

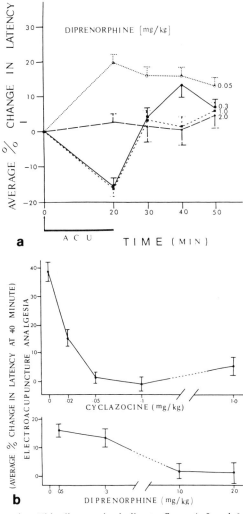

Fig. 7. a Effect of diprenorphine on EAA in mice. This diagram is similar to figure 4, 5 and 6. Diprenorphine was administered once (immediately before EA indicated by the arrow). Doses is indicated by the numerals 2, 1, 0.3 and 0.05 in mg/kg. **b** Dose-response curves showing that cyclazocine and diprenorphine reverses EAA in a dose-related manner in mice. Ordinate represents the EA effect (average % change of squeak latency at the 40 minute derived from Fig. 5 and 6). Abscissa indicates the dose concentration in mg/kg. Each point is mean of 15 mice. Upper curve shows the cyclazocine effect and lower curve shows the diprenorphine effect on EAA at various doses

4. More direct support of the acupuncture-endorphin hypothesis was obtained in 1977 when Sjolund, Terenius, and Erickson [29] reported that transcutaneous electroacupuncture (TE) on the lower lumbar spine (segmental TE) in humans elevated the lumber cerebrospinal fluid (CSF) endorphins (fraction 1) concentrations, while TE to nonsegmental TE did not. This "fraction" endorphin extract was subsequently found to cross react with dynorphin antigens (Terenius, personal com-

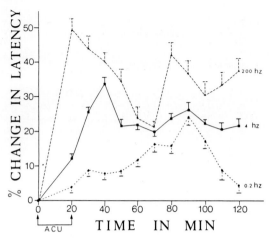

Fig. 8. Electroacupuncture analgesia induced by three different frequencies (200, 4 nd 0.2 Hz) of electrical stimulation. Ordinate shows average percentage change in latency to squeak as compared to zero time pretreatment control values. Positive values denote analgesia. Abscissa shows the time of measurements. Top line shows EA effect induced by 200 Hz. Middle line shows EA effect induced by 4 Hz. Bottom line shows EA effect induced by 0.2 Hz. Arrows indicate the time of E.A. Bars indicate standard error. Each point is the mean of 15 mice

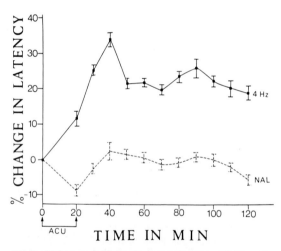

Fig. 9. Naloxone inhibits electroacupuncture (EA) analgesia which is induced by 4 Hz electrical stimulation. Coordinates same as Fig. 4. Upper line shows EA (at 4 Hz) effect on saline (0.9%) injected mice. Lower line shows EA effect on naloxone (1 mg/kg) injected mice. Injections were done twice: immediately before and after EA (at 0 and 20 minutes). Bars show standard errors. Arrows indicate the time of EA. Each point represents the mean of 15 mice

126

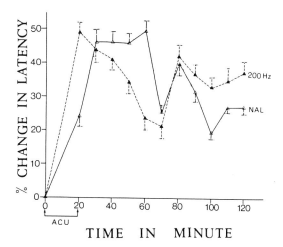

Fig. 10. Naloxone does not reverse the electroacupuncture (EA) effect at high frequency (200 Hz) stimulation. Coordinates same as Fig. 4. Dashed line (200 Hz) indicates EA in saline injected mice. Solid line (Nal) indicate EA in naloxone injected mice. Injections were given twice: immediately before and after EA. Arrows indicate the time of EA. Bars indicate standard errors. Each point is the mean of 15 mice

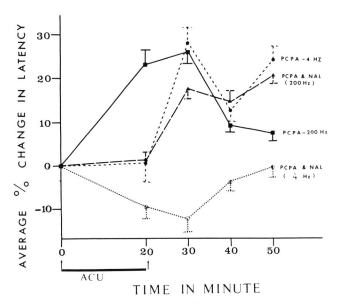

Fig. 11. Parachlorophenylalanine partially blocks high frequency (200 Hz) EA analgesia but not 4 Hz EA effect. Coordinates same as Fig. 4. 'PCPA-200 Hz' indicates high frequency EA treatment in PCPA treated mice. 'PCPA + Nal-(200 Hz)' indicates high frequency EA treatment in PCPA and naloxone treated mice. Treatment in PCPA treated mice. 'PCPA + Nal-(4 Hz)' indicates low frequency EA treatment in PCPA and naloxone injected mice. PCPA was injected 3 days before the experiment. Each point is the mean of 15 mice. Bars show standard error. Arrows indicate the beginning and end of EA and also the injections of naloxone or saline

127

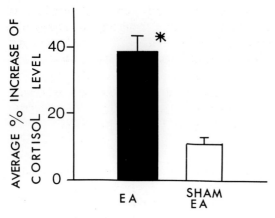

Fig. 12. The effect of electroacupuncture (EA) on blood cortisol level of horses. Ordinates indicate the average % increase of cortisol levels. Solid column indicates the average % increase of cortisol level of 15 horses after EA. Open column indicates the average % increase of blood cortisol level after sham EA in 15 horses. Bars indicate S. E. Star indicates statistical significance. EA significantly increases blood cortisol levels in horses

munication). Since dynorphin is found in the dorsal root ganglia [12], it was hypothesized that acupuncture can induce a local segmental release of endorphin (presumably dynorphin), which may then presynaptically inhibit the release of substance P. Substance P has been identified as one of the several potential neurotransmitters within primary nociceptive afferent neurons, whose cell bodies are located in the dorsal root ganglia. This substance is released at the central synapses of some primary afferent neurons following electrical stimulation of their high-threshold (C-fiber) axon. This release is blocked when morphine is applied in concentrations known to elicit analgesia: Han [17] further demonstrated that injection of dynorphin antibodies into rat spinal cord CSF inhibited EA in the 15–128 Hz frequency range. He speculated, therefore, that dynorphin mediated EA analgesia at the level of the spinal cord in this frequency range.

Tsou and colleagues [31] also found that EA caused an increase of endorphin (Fraction 1) levels in the cisternal CSF in rabbits; Zhang [35] demonstrated that fraction 1 endorphin release was elevated in the PAG of rabbits after acupuncture treatment. However, H. Akil has shown that injecting dynorphin into the PAG or ventricular CSF produces no analgesic effect in rats (personal communication), and thus the full role of dynorphin as a analgesic substance remains unclear.

Still, all the above results suggest that acupuncture releases endorphins into the CSF at several levels of the adding weight to the acupuncture-endorphin hypothesis.

5. It was demonstrated that D-phenylalanine and D-leucine produced naloxone-reversible analgesia in humans and mice [4, 5, 11]. It was postulated that these D-amino acids protected the endorphins from enzymatic degradation. Recent biochemical evidence supports this hypothesis; D-phenylalanine and D-leucine can cross the blood-brain barrier [21] and inhibit enkephalinases (demonstrated in guinea pig ileum assays [13]; It was then found [6] that combining these D-amino

128

acids and EA treatments produced analgesia in a greater number of mice in a test cohort than that produced by either treatment alone. Presumably, in keeping with the acupuncture endorphin hypothesis, EA released endorphins which were then protected from enzymatic degradation by the action of the D-amino acids.

6. It has been shown that hypophysectomy abolishes EA analgesia [1] and also that dexamethasone, which is known to inhibit the release of pituitary ACTH and β-endorphin, along with 2% saline treatment which depletes pituitary endorphin, all reduce EA analgesia [7]. These findings suggest that pituitary endorphin is at least partially involved in mediating EA analgesia. It has also been reported that hypophysectomy inhibits morphine analgesia (Katz 1980) and naloxone hyper-algesia [14]. This indicates that the pituitary is normally required for opiate analgesia. Finally, an indirect experiment indicated that EA may release endorphin and ACTH together into the blood, since plasma cortisol levels were elevated after EA analgesia in horses (7, 15) Fig. 12.

Evidently then, the acupuncture-endorphin hypothesis appears to implicate the existence of a highly complex neuroendocrine system for the mediation of EA analgesia (and by extension, for endogenous pain control). By integrating all the experimental data presented so far an internally consistent neurophysiological model for such a system can be proposed, but first another set of experimental data that implicates yet other complexities in the system must be considered. This set of data relates to the role of monoamines in EA analgesia.

Experimental Data Suggesting a Serotonin-Dependent System Mediating Electroacupuncture Analgesia

1. The raphe-serotonin descending inhibition system was first demonstrated by Shen and co-workers in 1975. They found that lesioning the dorsolateral fasciculus (DLF) completely abolished acupuncture analgesia in rabbits [27, 28]. In 1976, Du and Chao [10] showed that lesioning the raphe magnus also inhibited acupuncture analgesia. This result was repeated by McLennan [20], who showed that both electrical and chemical lesions of the raphe nucleus reduced EA in rabbits and in rats.

Injection of 5,6-dihydroxytryptamine (a chemical that destroys serotonin nerve endings) into the raphe nucleus inhibited EA analgesia [9]. Similarly, as described previously microinjection of naloxone into the PAG partially reversed EA analgesia [35]. Thus it is suggested that the raphe-DLF-serotonin system is linked in series to the enkephalinergic neurons in the raphe nucleus and PAG. (However, part of the PAG-EA analgesia effect may bypass the brain stem enkephalin system, as was previously suggested i.e., the PAG may be activated directly by the hypothalamus or the pituitary.)

In addition to 5,6-dihydroxytryptamine, many other chemicals that either deplete or antagonize the effects of brain serotonin have also been shown to abolish or reduce EA analgesia, while drugs that enhance the serotonin level in the CNS have been shown to increase EA analgesia [6, 16, 19]. These data all point to an important role of serotonin in EA analgesia. The results are presented in Table 1.

Table 1. Results of Acupuncture Research. Summary of monoaminergic drugs on EAA at 200 Hz. (Cheng R. 1981, Ph. D. Thesis)

Drug	Net Functional Change			EAA
1. TBZ	S↓	D↓	N↓	↓*
2. PCPA	S↓			↓*
3. AMPT		D↓	N↓	↓
4. Disulfiram	S↑		N↓	↑a
5. TBZ+5HTP	S↑	D↓	N↓	↑a
6. TBZ+L-DOPA	S↓	D↑	N↓	R (Partial)
7. PCPA+5HTP	Normal			Ra
8. AMPT+L-DOPA (1 hr)		D↑	N↓	R
9. AMPT+L-DOPA (2 hrs.)		D↓	N↑	R (Partial)
10. 5HTP	S↑			↑a
11. L-DOPA		D↑		↑
12. Probenecid	S↑	D↑		↑a
13. Apomorphine		D↑		↓
14. Cinanserin	S↓			↓a
15. Haloperidol		D↓		↓
16. Pimozide		D↓		→
17. Yohimbine			N↓	↓

S = Serotonin, D = Dopamine, N = Norepinephrine; R = Recovery of EAA after replacement drugs; TBZ = tetrabenazine; PCPA = parachloro-phenylalanine; AMPT = alpha-methyl-paratyroxine; 5HTP = DL-5-hydroxytryptophan; L-Dopa = L-3,4-dihydroxyphenylalaninmethylester.
a only the data related to serotonin gave consistent EAA results

2. Another important piece of evidence in support of the EA-serotonin hypothesis is that serotonin and its catabolite SHIAA were found to be elevated in the CSF [34], raphe nucleus and locus ceruleus [16, 32], spinal cord [16], and in the whole brain [16, 19]. During EA analgesia. The above-mentioned elevation of serotonin and its metabolite was positively correlated to the extent of EA analgesia, higher levels occurring with greater EA analgesia. Han [16] further demonstrated that the serotonin content and its turnover rate increased in the telencephalon, diencephalon, brain stem, and spinal cord after 1 h of EA treatment in rats. They also observed that certain areas of the CNS behaved differently in response to the same EA stimulation. There was a marked increase in serotonin synthesis in the lower brain stem and spinal cord but a marked increase of serotonin turnover in the diencephalon and telencephalon; they concluded from this that the forebrain might also play an important role in serotonin-mediated EA analgesia.
3. Iontophoretically applied serotonin or norepinephrine was found to inhibit the response of dorsal horn cells evoked by nociceptive stimulation; intrathecal application of these same chemicals in the spinal cord also produced a profound analgesia in rats, rabbits, and cats [33]. These results suggest the existence of descending systems which may modify spinal sensory processing by means of serotonin or norepinephrine.
4. Restating a finding described earlier Cheng and Pomeranz [2] demonstrated that while low-frequency (4 Hz) EA analgesia might be mediated by endorphins, high-frequency (200 Hz) EA analgesia might be mediated by a separate, serotonin-dependent system; the evidence for the existence of these dual systems was that the 4-Hz EA analgesia was partially reduced only by PCPA, the serotonin synthe-

Table 2. Results of Acupuncture Research (Cheng R. 1981, Ph. D. Thesis)

Treatment	Action	EAA (4 Hz)	EAA (200 Hz)
1 Hypophysectomy*	Deplete pituitary beta-endorphin	↓	ND
2 Dexamethasone	Inhibit beta-endorphin release	(partial) ↓	ND
3 2% saline feeding	Deplete pituitary endorphin	↓	ND
4 Type I opiate antagonists (i) Levo-naloxone (ii) Naltrexone (iii) Cyclazocine (iv) Diphrenorphine	Block type I opiate receptors	↓	ND
5 Dextro-naloxone	Inactive isomer	→	ND
6 D-Leucine and D-Phenylalanine	May enhance endorphins	↑	ND
7 Two EA treatments at 3 hrs apart	Cumulative effect	↑	ND
8 Morphine addicted mice during withdrawal	Addiction	↑	ND
9 PCPA	Deplete 5-HT	→	↓
10 Cinanserin	5-HT receptor blocker	ND	↓
11 5-HTP	5-HT precursor	ND	↑

Key: ↓ reduce EAA; ↑ increase EAA; → no effect on EAA; ND = not done

sis inhibitor. Similarly, Han [16] found that naloxone only partly blocked EA analgesia in rats. When the rats were injected with PCPA, again EA analgesia was only partly reduced. However, when the investigators combined naloxone and PCPA treatments together, EA analgesia, was completely abolished. This supports the Cheng and Pomeranz evidence for the existence of dual systems mediating EA analgesia, one dependent on endorphin and the other on serotonin [2].

Zhang [35] found that "moderate EA analgesia" (7.5–8.0 mA) was readily reversed by naloxone alone in rabbits, a result that would seem to contradict the studies [16] in which naloxone alone was insufficient to abolish EA analgesia. However, when Zhang et al. used "super strength EA analgesia (12.5–15.0 mA), they too could no longer reverse EA analgesia with naloxone alone. One explanation for these results is that the higher current stimulations (Han [16, 17] had used 5.0 mA in their studies, which is very high in comparison with the 0.1 mA threshold of Aβ fibers) may activate, in addition to the "normal" endorphin-dependent system, a second stress-induced analgesia which would be mediated by the non-endorphin system; low-intensity stimulation (nonnoxious) may activate only the endorphin-dependent system. In contrast, the Cheng and Pomeranz study [2] indicates that the non-endorphin system can also be activated by a low-intensity, non-noxious current (they used 0.1–0.2 mA impulse of 1-mS duration), provided one

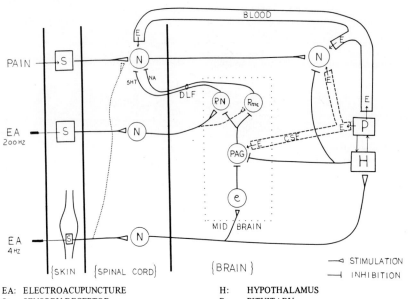

EA: ELECTROACUPUNCTURE
S: SENSORY RECEPTOR
N: INTERNEURON
e: ENKEPHALINERGIC NEURON
E: ENDORPHIN (β-ENDORPHIN or DYNORPHIN)
NA: NORADRENALINE

H: HYPOTHALAMUS
P: PITUITARY
PAG: PERIAQUEDUCTAL GRAY
RN: RAPHE NUCLEUS
RMC: RETICULAR MAGNOCELLAR NUCLEUS
DLF: DORSOLATERAL FUNICULUS

Fig. 13. At low frequency (4 Hz), EA may stimulate the midbrain (PAG) to release enkephalins which will indirectly stimulate the raphe nucleus (RN) and /or reticular magnocellular nucleus (Rmc) to send a descending inhibition on the spinal cord pain cells. Serotonin and noradrenaline are probably the neurotransmitters involved in the RN and Rmc systems respectively. In parallel, EA may also stimulate the hypothalamus and pituitary to release beta-endorphin or dynorphin. The pituitary endorphins may either go through the blood-brain barrier or backflow to the hypothalamus or CSF and bind to the opiate receptors in the spinal cord and the brain. In addition, low frequency (4 Hz) EA may cause the segmental release of endorphins from the spinal cord interneurons and bind to the opiate receptors in the pain transmission cells. High frequency (200 Hz) EA appears to stimulate directly the RN and Rmc descending inhibitory systems, bypassing the endorphin system

stimulated with high frequencies (they used 200 Hz); in their study, they could also trigger the endorphin system independently with low-intensity current of low frequency.

An Integrated Neurophysiological Model of Electroacupuncture Analgesia Is Proposed

Table 2 summarizes most of the data discussed in this article. From these data, a model of EA analgesia was constructed, which is presented in Fig. 13. Details of this model are further emphasized in Fig. 14 and 15, which isolate the postulated two pain-controlling systems from each other; these are the endorphin-dependent system and the serotonin-dependent system.

Briefly, it is proposed that low-frequency (4-Hz) EA stimulates the sensory receptors in deep muscle causing the midbrain PAG to release enkephalins. These

132

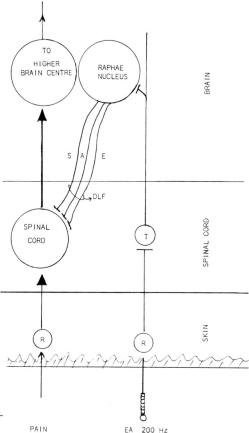

Fig. 14. Mechanism of high frequency electroacupuncture analgesia

PAIN   EA   200 Hz

enkephalins in turn activate the raphe nucleus (RN) and/or the reticular magno-cellular nucleus (RMC), which then send descending inhibitory signals along the DLF to the spinal cord; the RN-DLF pathway may use serotonin as its neuro-transmitter, while the RMC-DLF pathway may use norepinephrine. In the spinal cord the descending serotonergic and/or norepinephrinergic fibers would synapse with local enkephalinergic interneurons and activate (or disinhibit) these cells, leading to the release of enkephalins; these enkephalins may exert presynaptic inhibitory control over incoming substance P-containing primary afferent fibers concerned with pain transmission (Jessell and Iverson cellular model 1977). In parallel with this, low-frequency (4-Hz) EA may also stimulate the release of β-endorphin from the hypothalamus. These hypothalamic endorphin neurons project to different areas of the brain (e.g., PAG, periventricular nucleus of the thalamus, nucleus accumbens, amygdala) where they may release their β-endorphins and produce central pain relief. The EA-stimulated hypothalamus may also produce a releasing factor to stimulate the release of pituitary endorphins, and ACTH. These pituitary endorphins could then be released into the systemic circulation and be redistributed back to the brain and spinal cord by passing through

133

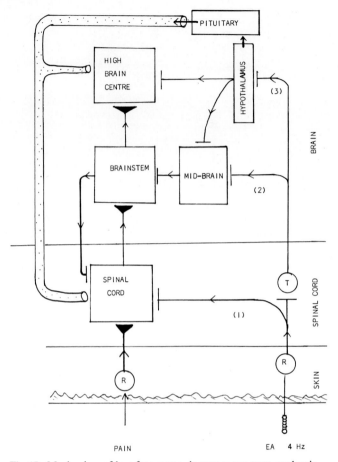

Fig. 15. Mechanism of low frequency electroacupuncture analgesia

the blood-brain barrier; at these locations they would bind to opiate receptors, causing analgesia. Low-frequency (4-Hz) EA may additionally cause segmental release of endorphins from the spinal cord interneurons and bind to the opiate receptors in the pain transmission cells, producing analgesia by presynaptic inhibition (suppressing the release of substance P). High-frequency (200-Hz) EA may activate sensory nerves and directly stimulate the DLF-serotonin/norepinephrine descending inhibitory systems, bypassing the PAG-endorphin system.

In summary, this model describes three anatomical levels of EA analgesia (Fig. 15):

1. Endorphin (dynorphin) release in the spinal cord would cause segmental or localized pain relief.

2. Activation of the midbrain and brain stem would induce a regional analgesia through the enkephalin-DLF-serotonin system. That is, EA to one part of the body would produce analgesia over a wide surface area which can be far removed from the site at which EA is applied. This can be understood if one

134

accepts the hypothesis advanced by Mayer et al. (1971) and Liesbeskind et al. (1973) that there exists a regional (Humunculus) mapping in the midbrain, whereby stimulation of a certain midbrain area will cause analgesia in a certain part of the body (e.g., in humans, stimulation of the first dorsal interosseous muscle in the hand produces analgesia in the facial area).

3. Activation of the hypothalamus and the pituitary would produce a generalized increase in the pain threshold. This effect would be mediated by the release of endorphins and ACTH into the systemic circulation; the endorphins so released would act via the pain-modulating systems already described while the ACTH would stimulate the release of cortisol, which would tend to reduce inflammation.

It is proposed that EA may stimulate the above levels individually, in part or all three together, resulting in different degrees of analgesia (as is observed in clinical practice). Higher analgesia and better clinical results can be obtained if acupuncture is done properly.

References

1. Cheng RSS (1977) Electroacupuncture effect on cat spinal cord neurons and conscious mice: A new hypothesis is proposed. M. Sc. Thesis, Zoology, University of Toronto
2. Cheng RSS, Pomeranz B (1979 a) Electroacupuncture analgesia could be mediated by at least two pain-relieving mechanisms; endorphin and non-endorphin systems. Life Sci 25, 1957-1962
3. Cheng RSS, Pomeranz B (1979 b) Correlation of genetic difference in endorphin systems with analgesic effects of d-amino acids in mice. Brain Res 177: 583-587
4. Cheng RSS, Pomeranz B (1980 a) Electroacupuncture analgesia is mediated by stereospecific opiate receptors and is reversed by antagonists of type I receptors. Life Sci 26: 631-639
5. Cheng RSS, Pomeranz B (1980 b) Monoaminergic mechanisms of electroacupuncture analgesia. Brain Res 215: 77-93
6. Cheng RSS, Pomeranz B (1980 c) A combined treatment with D-amino acids and electroacupuncture produces a greater analgesia than either treatment alone: naloxone reverses these effects, Pain 8, 231-236
7. Cheng RSS, Pomeranz B, Yu G (1979 a) Dexamethasone partially reduces and 2% saline treatment abolished electroacupuncture analgesia: These findings implicate pituitary endorphins. Life Sci 24: 1481-1486
8. Cheng RSS, McKibbin L, Buddha R, Pomeranz B (1980 c) Electroacupuncture elevates blood cortisol levels in naive horse; sham treatment has no effect. Intern J Neurosci 10: 95-97
9. Chiang CY, Tu HX, Chao YF, PAI YH, Ku HK, Cheng JK, Shang HY, Yang FY (1979) Effect of electrolytic or intracerebral injections of 5,6-dihydroxtrytamine in raphe nuclei on acupuncture analgesia in rats. Chin Med J 92: 129-136
10. Du HJ, Chao YF (1976) Localization of central structure involved in descending inhibitory effect of acupuncture on viscero-somatic reflex discharges. Scientia Sinica 19: 137-148
11. Ehrenpreis S, Balagot RC, Comathy J, Myles S (1978) Naloxone reversible analgesia in mice, produced by inhibitors of enkephalin. In second world congress on pain, vol 1, Montreal, p 260
12. Goldstein A, Tachibana S, Lowney LI, Hunkapiller M, Hood L (1979) Dynorphin-(1-13) An extra-ordinarily potent opioid peptide. Proc Natl Acad Sci, USA, 76: 6666-6670
13. Greenberg J, Kubota K, Ehrenpreis S (1980) Bioassay of brain enkephalinases: Inhibition by d-phenylalanine (DPA) and other substances producing analgesia in mice. Fed Proc 39: 606
14. Grevert P, Baizman ER, Goldstein A (1978) Naloxone effects on a nociceptive response of hypophysectomized and adrenalectomized mice. Life Sci 23: 723-728

15. Guillemin R, Vargo T, Rossier J, Minick S, Ling H, Rivier C, Vale W, Bloom R (1977) B-endorphin and adrenocorticotropin are secreted concomitantly by the pituitary gland. Science 197: 1367-1369
16. Han CS, Chou PH, Lu CC, Lu LH, Yang TH, Jen MF (1979) The role of central 5-hydroxytryptamine in acupuncture analgesia. Scientia Sinica 22: 91-104
17. Han JS, Xie GX (1984) Dynorphin: Important mediator for electroacupuncture analgesia in the spinal cord of the rabbit. Pain 18: 367-377
18. Katz RJ (1979) Hypophysectomy reduces Behavioral activation to morphine in the rat. Behavioral physiology
19. Kim KC, Han YF, Yu LP, Feng J, Wang FS, Zhang ZD, Change AZ, Shen MP, Lu YY (1979) Role of brain serotonergic and catecholaminergic systems in acupuncture analgesia. Acta Physiol Sinica 31: 121-131
20. McLennen H, Gilfillan K, Heap Y (1977) Some pharmacological observations on the analgesia induced by acupuncture in rabbits. Pain 3: 229-238
21. Okafor C, Mosnaim AD, Ehrenpreis S (1980) Uptake of D-phenylalanine (DPA) by mouse brain: Correlation with analgesic activity. Fed Proc 39: 386
22. Peets J, Pomeranz B (1978) CXBK mice dificient in opiate receptors show poor electroacupuncture analgesia. Nature 273: 675-676
23. Pomeranz B, Cheng R (1979) Suppression of noxious responses in single neurons of cat spinal cord by electroacupuncture and its reversal by the opiate antagonist naloxone. Exp Neurol 64: 327-341
24. Pomeranz BH, Cheng R, Law P (1977) Acupuncture Reduces electrophysiological and behavioral responses to noxious stimuli: pituitary is implicated. Exp Neurol 54: 172-178
25. Pomeranz BH, Chiu D (1976) Naloxone blocks acupuncture analgesia and causes hyperalgesia: Endorphin is implicated. Life Sci 19: 1757-1762
26. Pomeranz B, Paley D (1979) Electroacupuncture hypalgesia is mediated by afferent nerve impulses: an electrophysiological study in mice. Exp Neurol 66: 398-402
27. Shen E, Ma WH, Lau C (1978) Involvement of descending on the splanchnically evoked potential in the orbital cortex of cat. Scientia Sinica 21: 677-685
28. Shen E, Tsai T, Lau C (1975) Supraspinal participation in the inhibitory effect of acupuncture on viscerosomatic reflex discharges. Chin Med J 1: 431-440
29. Sjolund B, Terenius L, Eriksson M (1977) Increased cerebrospinal fluid levels of endorphins after electroacupuncture. Acta Physiol Scand 100: 382-384
30. Takeshige C, Kamada T, Oka K, Hisamitsu M (1978) The relationship between midbrain neurons (periaqueduct centrol gray and midbrain reticular formation) and acupuncture analgesia. Animal hypnosis. Second world congress on pain (abstract) vol 1, Montreal, p 156
31. Tsou K, Wu SH, Wan FS, Ji XQ, Chang TS, Lo ES, Yi CC (1979) Increased levels of endorphins in the cisternal cerebrospinal fluid of rabbits in acupuncture analgesia. Acta Physiologica Sinica 31: 371-376
32. Tung HW, Chiang CH, Fu LW (1978) Changes in monoamine fluorescence intensity in the rats midbrain raphe nuclei and locus coerulus in the process of acupuncture analgesia. Acta Biochem at Biophysica Sinica 10: 119-125
33. Yaksh TL, Wilson PR (1979) Spinal serotonin terminal system mediates antinociception. J of Pharmacol and Exp Therap 208: 446-453
34. Yi CC, Lu TH, Wu SH, Tsou K (1977) A study of the release of H(3)-5-hydroxytrytamine from brain during acupuncture and morphin analgesia. Scientia Sinica 20: 113-124
35. Zhang AZ, Pan X, Chen J, Mo W, Sun F (1979) Endorphins and acupuncture analgesia. In: National symposia of acupuncture and moxibustion and acupuncture anaesthesia. Beijing, China, p 32

Neurophysiological Mechanisms of Acupuncture Analgesia in Experimental Animal Models

Jin Mo Chung

Marine Biomedical Institute and Departments of Anatomy and Neuroscience and of Physiology and Biophysics, University of Texas Medical Branch, 200 University Boulevard, Galveston, Texas 77550, USA

Introduction

Acupuncture and transcutaneous electrical nerve stimulation (TENS) are two different procedures which result in analgesia by stimulation of peripheral tissues. Acupuncture, using either the traditional technique of manual rotation of needles [3, 35, 36, 62] or electroacupuncture [2, 3, 36], has been used successfully as an anesthetic [5, 32] and as a treatment for chronic pain [6, 24, 42, 61]. TENS has been widely used in the West to produce analgesia clinically, as well as in experimental animal models [31, 44, 50, 56, 63, 73]. Like TENS, the effects of acupuncture appear to be due to the activation of peripheral nerve fibers [11, 22, 25, 43, 53, 59, 69]. Although acupuncture is effective in producing analgesia, the reported effectiveness varies greatly between studies. For example, in studies performed in the West alone, analgesia produced by acupuncture ranges from a mild effect to the one spectacular enough to allow performance of open heart surgery [32]. Not only the effectiveness but also the methodology of stimulation varies between laboratories. For example, frequency of stimulation for electroacupuncture ranges from several pulses per second [2, 26] to 10 KHz [43, 48]. The lack of a standard method of application and the inconsistency of the effects between studies are primarily due to incomplete understanding of the mechanisms of acupuncture (and TENS) analgesia, which greatly hampers further development of the technique.

In an attempt to study the mechanisms of acupuncture and TENS analgesia, experimental animal models were developed. Using these models, some important factors determining analgesic effectiveness were investigated. The basic approach has been electrophysiological recording of neuronal activity in the spinal cord, which can be used as a nociceptive index, and its modulation by electrical stimulation applied directly to a peripheral nerve in an anesthetized animal.

Experimental Animal Models

Development of Experimental Cat Model. It is important to study the mechanisms of acupuncture and TENS for technical improvement of the analgesic procedures as well as for improving understanding of the pain control mechanisms in general. To study the underlying mechanisms, it is vitally important to develop a good experimental animal model. I attempted to develop animal models which permit not only a wide range of experimental manipulations but also the measurement of objective indices that reflect levels of pain.

137

First developed was an experimental cat model using the flexion reflex as the pain index. The cat was anemically decerebrated by ligating the carotid arteries bilaterally and the basilar artery under ketamine anesthesia. The flexion reflex was recorded as a compound action potential in the hamstring nerve while evoking the reflex by electrically stimulating the sural nerve with an intensity high enough to activate unmyelinated C fibers (20 V, 0.5 ms). The flexion reflex consisted of two components: early and late. The early and late components have latencies of about 10 and 200 ms and durations of about 10 ms and 1 s, respectively [29]. To test the viability of the flexion reflex as a pain index in this preparation, its sensitivity to systemically injected morphine was examined [17]. Although IV injection of morphine tended to depress the early component, the results were highly variable between experiments. The late component was reliably depressed by systemic injection of morphine in a dose-related fashion. The late component was very sensitive to IV injections of morphine: it was depressed to 50% and 25% of the original size with doses of 1 and 2 mg/kg, respectively. Furthermore, this depressant effect by morphine was reversed by a small dose of naloxone (0.05–0.1 mg/kg). From the results of these studies, in conjunction with the fact that the flexion reflex has classically been known as a common nociceptive reflex [65], I felt that the late component of the flexion reflex could be used as a reasonably good pain index.

Using this model (flexion reflex in anemically decerebrated cat), testing of the analgesic effect of acupuncture was begun. Electroacupuncture was performed using a 28-gauge hyperdermic needle on the St.36 Zusanli point in the lateral upper tibial region of the ipsilateral hindlimb (tibialis anterior muscle) [53]. Stimulation was applied with high intensity pulses (20 V, 2 ms) repeated at a rate of 2 Hz for 1 h. This electroacupuncture procedure produced depression of the late component of the flexion reflex to less than half the size of the prestimulus control, which is comparable to the effect produced by systemic injection of morphine 1 mg/kg. The depression of the flexion reflex produced by electroacupuncture was reversed by a systemic injection of naloxone. When all peripheral nerves (except the sural nerve) in the ipsilateral hindlimb were cut, the effect of electroacupuncture was no longer observed, while direct electrical stimulation of the common peroneal nerve at the proximal end with the same stimulus parameters mimicked the effect of electroacupuncture. In these results, electroacupuncture applied in an experimental animal produced an analgesic effect which was apparently initiated by afferent nerve activity. The effect seems to be mediated by the release of opiate substances.

Since it is difficult to perform a quantitative analysis on recordings of compound action potentials, the model was then refined, based on the recording of the flexion reflex as single unit activity from motor axons [12]. The activity in single motor axons was recorded from filaments of the L7, S1, or S2 ventral roots in the cat. The reflex activity in the motor axons was elicited either by electrical stimulation of a hindlimb nerve or by natural forms of stimulation applied to the foot. As in recordings of compound action potentials, electrical stimulation of an afferent nerve elicited early and late components of the flexion reflex, the late component representing activation of Aδ and C afferent fibers. When natural forms of stimuli were applied to the foot, sustained activity in the motor axons could only

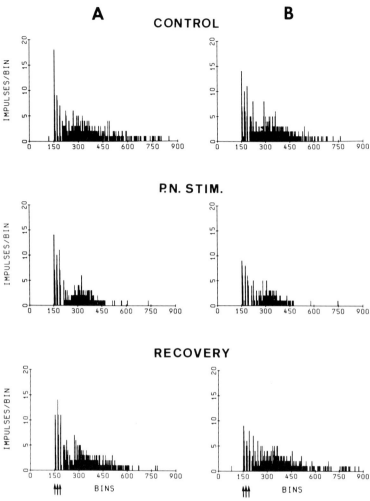

Fig. 1 A, B. Effects of peripheral nerve stimulation on the flexion reflex in a spinal cat. **A** Reflex was elicited by electrical stimulation of the common peroneal nerve *(upper histogram)*. Inhibition (to 52% of control) of the reflex was observed immediately after stimulation of the tibial nerve at a rate of 2 Hz for 15 min *(middle histogram)*. The reflex gradually recovered with time, reaching 101% of control 40 min after the termination of the stimulus *(lower histogram)*. **B** After the reflex recovered from the inhibition, another control reflex discharge was recorded *(upper histogram)*. Stimulation of the tibial nerve a second time produced a greater inhibition (to 41% of control, *middle histogram*). Then naloxone hydrochloride 0.05 mg/kg was given intravenously and the reflex recovered to 92% of control 10 min later *(lower histogram)*. All histograms were compiled from responses to 10 consecutive stimuli, and bin widths are 2 ms. *P. N. STIM.,* peripheral nerve stimulation. (Reproduced from [12])

be elicited by intense noxious mechanical or thermal stimuli. This fact reinforces the contention that the flexion reflex could be used as a pain index. Since the results of an earlier study indicated that the analgesic effects produced by electroacupuncture and direct peripheral stimulation are comparable [53], conditioning stimulation was applied to the common peroneal or tibial nerve at a suprathreshold intensity for C fibers at a rate of 2 Hz for 15 or 30 min. This produced an inhibition of the flexion reflex late discharges which outlasted the conditioning stimuli. Maximum inhibition on average was about 40% and 43% of the control reflex value in decerebrate and spinal cats, respectively. In decerebrate cats, the duration of inhibition varied from less than 10 min to over 1 h beyond termination of the conditioning stimuli, depending on the unit. However, inhibition lasted over 20 min for all units tested in spinal animals. The long-lasting inhibition of the flexion reflex was reversed by a systemic injection of naloxone hydrochloride (0.05 mg/kg). Figure 1 A shows an example of this analgesic effect recorded in the spinal cat and Fig. 1 B shows its reversal by naloxone.

Development of Experimental Monkey Model. Although the flexion reflex appears to be a good pain index, the reflex is a pain reaction (motor reflex) rather than a phenomenon related to pain perception per se. Therefore, it seems desirable to develop a model based on a more direct indicator of pain sensation such as the activity of nociceptive tract neurons. The spinothalamic tract (STT) is one of the best known nociceptive tracts in primates, including humans [40, 52, 71, 72]. Primate STT cells are well suited to transmit pain information to the brain since they respond well to various forms of noxious stimuli applied to the periphery [14, 23, 37]. Furthermore, various analgesic manipulations inhibit their activity [27, 28, 30]. Hence, it was decided to use the activity of monkey STT cells evoked by unmyelinated C fibers in the sural nerve as a pain index to test the analgesic effect produced by peripheral conditioning stimulation [13].

Identified STT cells were recorded from the lumbosacral spinal cord or intact, anesthetized monkeys. In addition, presumed STT cells were recorded from both unanesthetized/decerebrated, and decerebrated/spinal monkeys. Presumed STT cells were identified by antidromically activating them from the contralateral, ventral, lateral funiculus of the cervical spinal cord. Both C fiber activity evoked by electrical stimulation of the sural nerve and the activity evoked by noxious heat were greatly inhibited by repetitive conditioning stimuli applied either to the common peroneal or tibial nerve with a strong enough intensity for activation of C fibers at 2 Hz for 15 min. The inhibition was maintained during the period of conditioning stimulation and often outlasted it by 20–30 min as shown in Fig. 2. The inhibition of cells produced by peripheral nerve stimulation was observed in decerebrate and spinalized animals as well as in intact anesthetized monkeys, although the mean recovery time in the decerebrate group was faster. This indicates that anesthesis does not interfere with the inhibitory mechanisms. Furthermore, the presence of inhibition in spinalized animals suggest that the inhibition must depend in part on spinal cord neuronal circuitry.

Although direct peripheral nerve conditioning stimulation produced inhibition of STT-cell activity, it was interesting to try a commercially available TENS unit on a monkey to test clinical applicability. The C-fiber-evoked, STT-cell activity

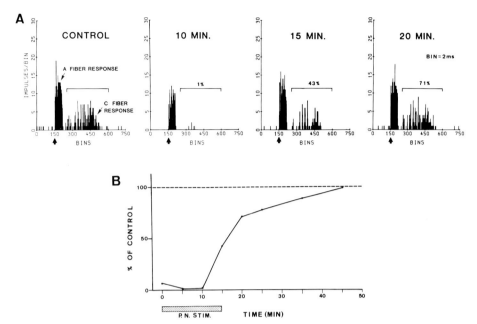

Fig. 2 A, B. Inhibition of a monkey spinothalamic tract cell produced by peripheral nerve stimulation. **A** Poststimulus time histograms showing *A-* and *C-fiber responses* following stimulation *(large arrow at bottom)* of the sural nerve. Histograms were formed from 10 consecutive stimuli. The C-fiber responses (indicated by *brackets*) were observed before, during, and after repetitive stimulation of the common peroneal nerve with an intensity suprathreshold for C fibers at 2 Hz for 15 min. The C-fiber responses were inhibited to 1%, 43%, and 71% of control value at 10 min during, immediately after, and 5 min after 15 min of conditioning stimulation, respectively. **B** The C-fiber evoked response was plotted to show the full time course of recovery. *P. N. STIM.,* peripheral nerve stimulation. (Reproduced from [13])

was compared before, during, and after application of TENS for 5 min while monitoring the current delivered by the TENS unit [41]. Application of TENS produced inhibition of C-fiber-evoked, STT-cell activity. Powerful inhibition of STT-cell activity occurred during application of TENS, and the inhibition gradually recovered after termination. Therefore, using this experimental monkey model, an analgesic effect was demonstrated not only by direct conditioning stimulation of a peripheral nerve but also by application of a commercially available TENS unit.

Animal Preparation. In these animal models, three different preparations were used: animals with intact brains and anesthetized with anesthetic drugs; unanesthetized, decerebrate animals; and unanesthetized, decerebrate/spinal animals. In most cases, the animal was prepared by performing a decerebration followed by a spinalization, after which the anesthetic drug could be discontinued. The spinal animal provides several advantages. First, the flexion reflex, a pain index which was recorded, is severely depressed in the presence of a common anesthetic drug [51]. While the flexion reflex is extremely unstable in unanesthetized/decerebrate preparations, it is strong and stable in spinal animals [12].

Second, analgesic mechanisms can be studied without the potential complications of anesthetic drugs. Third, the antinociceptive effect that was observed mainly depends on spinal mechanisms, as evidenced by the lack of a significant change of the observed effect after spinalization [13]. Fourth, although spinalization eliminates any potential contribution of supraspinal structures for the production of analgesic effects, it was thought important to study the spinal mechanisms first without the complication of supraspinal influences. After the spinal mechanisms are fully unveiled, the search can then be extended to supraspinal mechanisms.

Analgesic Stimulation. In these experimental animal models, a peripheral nerve was stimulated directly with electrical pulses (rather than application of acupuncture or TENS) because they are more controllable. Since both acupuncture and TENS are forms of peripheral nerve stimulation, direct stimulation of a peripheral nerve with proper parameters should mimic these procedures. To be able to manipulate with a variety of combinations of stimulus parameters, including a high enough intensity to activate C fibers, a model using an anesthetized and paralyzed animal was chosen. Partly because a behavioral pain index cannot be used in an anesthetized animal and partly to obtain an objective index, neuronal activity that reflects the level of pain was recorded as a pain index.

Components of Analgesic Effect

It is controversial as to whether or not the analgesia produced by acupuncture is naloxone reversible [4, 49, 58]. It has been reported that both TENS [67, 68] and electroacupuncture [9] with low-frequency stimulation produce naloxone-reversible analgesia, whereas high-frequency stimulation produces analgesia that is not naloxone reversible. However, Woolf et al. [74] were able to produce naloxone-reversible analgesia with high-frequency, percutaneous, nerve stimulation. Therefore, it is not clear whether or not the production of naloxone-reversible analgesia is stimulus-frequency dependent.

Results from this laboratory indicate that low-frequency stimulation of a peripheral nerve, in fact, produces both the naloxone-reversible and non-naloxone-reversible components of analgesia simultaneously [13, 15]. As shown in Fig. 2, analgesic effects in the monkey start to appear within a few seconds after the beginning of repetitive conditioning stimulation and gradually but rapidly build up so that the maximum effect can be seen within minutes. The maximum effect is generally maintained throughout the duration of stimulation. At the termination of the stimulation, the antinociceptive effect gradually fades away after dozens of minutes. When identical conditioning stimulation is repeated following systemic injection of naloxone, as shown in Fig. 3, no significant difference can be seen during stimulation, but recovery from the analgesic effect after termination of the stimulation occurs slightly but significantly faster. This phenomenon was interpreted as evidence indicating that the analgesic effect produced by peripheral conditioning stimulation consists of two different components, naloxone reversible and non-naloxone reversible.

142

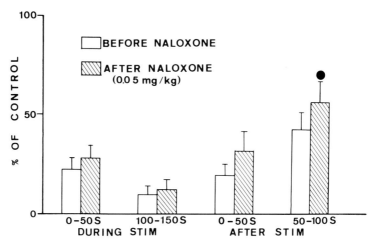

Fig. 3. Effect of naloxone on the inhibition produced by peripheral nerve stimulation in the monkey. After demonstrating good inhibition by repetitive conditioning stimulation of the tibial nerve for 5 min (intensity was suprathreshold for $A\delta$ fibers, and frequency was between 2 and 20 Hz, depending on the unit), the identical conditioning stimuli were repeated 5 min after intravenous injection of naloxone hydrochloride (0.05 mg/kg). Data were collected from 13 spinothalamic tract cells. The C-fiber evoked responses measured during the first 50 s of conditioning stimulation *(STIM)*, during the period between 100 and 150 s of conditioning stimulation, and during the first and second 50-s periods following termination of conditioning stimulation are expressed as a percentage of the average prestimulus control values. Each *bar* indicates 1 SEM. The *dot* represents a significantly ($P < 0.05$) different value from the one obtained before naloxone injection. (Reproduced from [15])

Figure 4 illustrates a hypothetical development and recovery of analgesia produced by peripheral nerve conditioning stimulation. The concept of this figure is based partly on personal experimental results and partly on an attempt to explain controversial published results from other laboratories. The analgesic effect produced by peripheral nerve conditioning stimulation is the summed effect of the naloxone-reversible and non-naloxone-reversible components. The non-naloxone-reversible component is much more powerful, develops quickly, and is short lasting. On the other hand, the naloxone-reversible component is weaker and develops slowly, but lasts for a long period of time. To be able to observe the naloxone-reversible component, the duration of the conditioning stimulation has to be long. During conditioning stimulation, the naloxone-reversible component is difficult to detect due to the dominance of the powerful non-naloxone-reversible component. However, at the tail end of the recovery period, it should be easy to detect the naloxone-reversible component if one employs a method that is sensitive enough. It is further hypothesized that the magnitude of each of the two components depends on multiple variables such as animal preparation (types of anesthesia, decerebration or spinalization, etc.), types of afferent nerves being stimulated, patterns of conditioning stimulation (frequency, patterned bursts, etc.), and species. Therefore, it is possible to observe, either completely or partially, naloxone-reversible or non-naloxone-reversible analgesia produced by peripheral nerve conditioning stimulation, depending on the time of observation, the type of

143

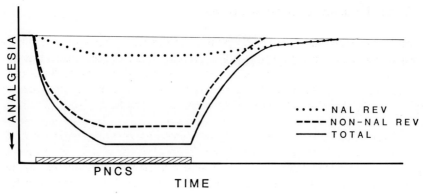

Fig. 4. A hypothetical diagram showing production of analgesia by peripheral nerve conditioning stimulation. The degree of analgesic effect is plotted (*downward,* greater analgesia) against time. The total analgesic effect is the sum of two components, naloxone-reversible *(NAL REV)* and non-naloxone-reversible *(NON-NAL REV)* analgesia. These two components are produced simultaneously in normal situations. However, some conditions may favor the production of one component while other conditions favor the other component. In general, the non-naloxone-reversible component is much more powerful than the naloxone-reversible component. The non-naloxone-reversible component develops quickly and lasts for only a short time. On the other hand, the naloxone-reversible component develops slowly and is long lasting. *PNCS,* a period of peripheral nerve conditioning stimulation

animal preparation used, and the method of conditioning stimulation. However, it is still not clear what the exact conditions are which favor the production of one or the other type of analgesia.

Although it is reasonably clear that the naloxone-reversible component is mediated by opiates, the chemical mediators for the non-naloxone-reversible component are not known. The tens of seconds required for the development of the non-naloxone-reversible component seem to be to slow for purelx electrical events. Attempts were made to interfere pharmacologically with this component [13], but none of the agents tested changed the inhibition to any appreciable degree. Drugs tested included GABA blockers (picrotoxin and bicuculline) and the glycine blocker strychnine, since these are well-known to have an action on spinal inhibitory mechanisms. Serotonin and catecholamine blockers (metergoline and phentolamine) were also tested since these monoamines have been implicated in acupuncture analgesia [29a]. It is possible that another known chemical agent, such as one of the neuropeptides other than enkephalin, or accumulation of K^+ [39] mediates the non-naloxone-reversible analgesia.

Although the chemical mediators are not known, this component is powerful and develops quickly, making it easy to study and allowing versatile experimental manipulations. Therefore, most of my subsequent work was focused mainly on the non-naloxone-reversible component of analgesia.

Some Factors Influencing Analgesic Effects

It is important to note that all the findings made in this laboratory concerning factors influencing analgesia are for non-naloxone-reversible analgesia (except in the cat studies described above), which is powerful but has a short onset latency and quick recovery. It is possible that the naloxone-reversible component is determined by completely different factors than those described here.

Size of Afferent Fibers that Produce Analgesia. Acupuncture analgesia is reported to be related to the activation of Aβ or group II fibers [3, 35, 59, 69], but evidence for this is not definitive. Woolf et al. [74] found that strong percutaneous stimulation which excited Aδ fibers elicited a more powerful analgesia than did weak stimulation. In addition, several conflicting reports appear in Chinese abstracts. Two groups of workers [8, 45] claimed that acupuncture analgesia is transmitted mainly by large A fibers, while another group [7] concluded that small fibers (including unmyelinated fibers) contribute more to the analgesia than do large fibers. Therefore it is not clear what size of afferent fibers triggers the peripheral nerve stimulation-produced analgesia.

In one study [15], the C-fiber-evoked, STT-cell activity was compared before, during, and after repetitive conditioning stimuli were applied to the tibial nerve for 5 min. As shown in Fig.5, very little analgesic effect was produced by the conditioning stimulation at a strength that was sufficient to activate most of the A$\alpha\beta$ fibers but none of the Aδ fibers of the tibial nerve. However, when the conditioning stimulus strength was increased to a level that activated many of the Aδ fibers, there was a powerful analgesic effect. When the strength of the conditioning stimulus was increased still further to include C fibers, the inhibition became even more powerful. Since the largest increment of the analgesic effect occurred when Aδ fibers were recruited, it can be concluded that the Aδ fiber group is the most important for producing the analgesic effect, although significant additional effects were also produced by the A$\alpha\beta$ and C fiber groups. When TENS was applied in the experimental monkey model while monitoring the current delivered by a commercially available TENS unit, inhibition of C-fiber-evoked, STT-cell activity occurred only when the intensity of TENS exceeded the threshold of the Aδ fibers [41]. The result obtained from the cat experiment is consistent with the above findings [66]. Conditioning stimulation applied to the tibial nerve at an intensity that excites only A$\alpha\beta$ fibers produced weak inhibition of the flexion reflex; increasing intensity above the threshold for Aδ fibers produced much greater inhibition. Results of the above studies suggest that the critical afferent fiber group that triggers an analgesic effect upon activation is the Aδ fiber group.

Most Effective Stimulus Frequency. A wide range of frequencies has been used to produce analgesic effects by peripheral nerve stimulation. It ranges from several pulses per second [2, 26] to 10 KHz [43, 48]. Although all of these stimulation frequencies seem to produce analgesia, it is not known which is the most effective. For low-frequency stimulation, Cheng and Pomeranz [9] reported that 4 Hz gives a better result than 0.2 Hz. Also while 4 Hz analgesia was blocked by naloxone, 100 Hz was not. Eriksson et al. [21] used short trains of pulses (100 Hz internal fre-

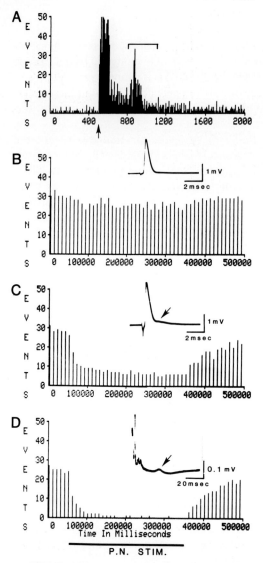

Fig. 5 A–D. Inhibition of a spinothalamic tract cell produced by peripheral nerve stimulation with graded strengths in the monkey. **A** The peristimulus time histogram was compiled after 10 consecutive stimuli (at the time indicated by *arrow*) applied to the sural nerve (bin width, 8 ms). The C-fiber evoked responses indicated by the *bracket* were used to form histograms in **B–D**. **B–D.** While collecting C-fiber evoked responses to test stimuli applied to the sural nerve every 10 s throughout the recording period, graded strengths of conditioning stimuli were applied to the tibial nerve at a frequency of 2 Hz for 5 min. Intensities of conditioning stimuli for *B, C,* and *D* were 2.3 times A$\alpha\beta$ fiber threshold, 20 times Aδ fiber threshold, and 3 times C fiber threshold, respectively. Volleys shown in *insets* were recorded from the tibial nerve 2 cm distal to the stimulating electrodes. *Arrows* in **C** and **D** indicate the Aδ and C waves, respectively. Bin widths in **B–D,** 2 s. (Reproduced from [15])

146

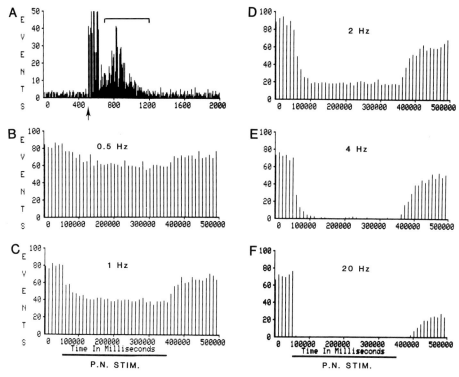

Fig. 6 A–F. Inhibition of a spinothalamic tract cell produced by peripheral nerve stimulation at different frequencies in the monkey. In **A** the evoked A and C responses are shown in a peristimulus time histogram which was compiled from 10 consecutive stimuli applied to the sural nerve at the time indicated by the *arrow* (bin width, 8 ms). The C-fiber evoked responses indicated by the *bracket* were used to form histograms in **B–F**. **B–F** Data collection was similar to that in Fig. 5, except that conditioning stimuli were delivered with a strength of 10 times Aδ fiber threshold and with the frequency indicated *above each histogram. P. N. STIM.,* peripheral nerve stimulation. (Reproduced from [15])

quency, 700-ms duration) repeated at a rate of 2 Hz to improve both the effectiveness of analgesia and the patient tolerance over either 100-Hz or 2-Hz fixed rate stimulation.

The results of personal study [41] confirmed this in that TENS with bursts of pulses at a low rate ("comfort bursts"; 3 bursts/s, 7 pulses/burst, internal frequency 85 Hz) was more effective in producing inhibition of STT-cell activity in the monkey than that with a fixed rate of high-frequency pulses (85 Hz) at a given intensity. However, when the different frequencies of fixed rates were compared, it was found that the higher the frequency, the more powerful was the analgesia which resulted within the range (0.5–20 Hz) tested [15]. In this study, the C-fiber-evoked, STT-cell activity was compared during conditioning stimuli of varying frequencies applied to the tibial nerve for 5 min. As shown in Fig. 6, the conditioning stimulus was set at a strength above threshold for Aδ fibers, and the stimulus frequency was varied from 0.5 to 20 Hz. There was weak inhibition with the frequency at 0.5 Hz, and the inhibition increased progressively as the stimulus frequency was increased. Stimulus frequency beyond 20 Hz could not be tested because the STT-cell activity is generally completely suppressed at 20 Hz, making further comparison difficult. Therefore, it seems likely that higher frequency stimulation is more effective than lower frequency in producing an analgesic effect within a reasonable range, at least for the non-naloxone-reversible component. (But frequencies above 4 Hz at intensities sufficient to activate Aδ fibers would cause intolerable muscle spasm due to tetanic contractions.)

Stimulation Point Specificity. Acupuncture can be applied to any of several hundred known acupuncture points all over the body. It has been reported that the application of acupuncture to a particular point is critical for analgesia to develop in a given region of the body [18, 26, 38, 69]. Although the old Chinese acupuncture theory of a hypothetical system of energy channels or meridians was considered the basis for acupuncture specificity [3, 36], the current scientific explanation of acupuncture does not support this. Since acupuncture is a form of peripheral nerve stimulation, the exact point of stimulation should not make much difference as long as the innervating nerve is stimulated effectively. Furthermore, particular acupuncture points on the body are believed to exert effects on specific areas some distance away from the points [10, 70]. However, the result of a carefully controlled experiment showed that acupuncture in a given point decreased pain sensitivity by the same degree in "target" and "non-target" areas [46]. On the other hand, TENS is generally most effective when electrodes are placed within the painful dermatome [21, 44].

To test stimulation point specificity in this experimental animal model, conditioning stimulation was applied to nerves innervating different parts of the body [15]. The most effective nerve in producing inhibition of activity of STT cells recorded from the monkey lumbosacral spinal cord was the ipsilateral tibial nerve. The contralateral sciatic nerve, the ipsilateral median nerve, and the contralateral median nerve were less effective, in that order. This result suggests that the inhibition of STT-cell activity produced by peripheral nerve stimulation is segmentally organized. A similar result was obtained by applying TENS with a commercially available TENS unit [41]. Furthermore, no systematic difference in analgesic effect produced by stimulation of the tibial or common peroneal nerve has been noted [13]. Therefore, no evidence for stimulation point specificity for the production of analgesia was seen in these studies, at least for the non-naloxone-reversible component. It is possible that the powerful non-naloxone-reversible analgesic effect produced here is equivalent to the TENS effect which is reportedly organized segementally without precise stimulation point specificity [31, 34, 56].

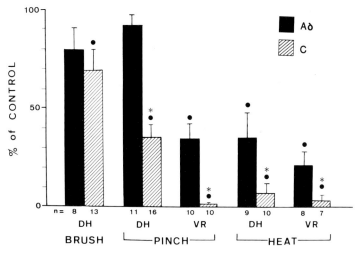

Fig. 7. Effect of peripheral conditioning stimulation on the activity of dorsal horn cells *(DH)* and ventral root motor axons *(VR)* evoked by mechanical and thermal stimuli in the spinal cat. The activity of the dorsal horn cells was evoked by application of innocuous mechanical (repetitive brushing with a camel's hair brush), noxious mechanical (pinching a fold of the skin with a pair of serrated forceps), and noxious heat (application of noxious thermal stimulation with a contact petier thermode) stimuli applied to the skin within the receptive fields. The reflex activity in motor axons could only be evoked by noxious stimuli. The evoked activity obtained immediately after conditioning stimulation of the tibial nerve at 2 Hz for 5 min was compared with the prestimulus control evoked activity. Data are expressed as mean percentage of the control value (*bars* indicate SEM). *Dots* indicate values significantly different from the controls. *Asterisks* indicate values significantly different from those obtained after conditioning stimulation at $A\delta$ fiber strength. Note that the dorsal horn cell activity evoked by pinching was inhibited more than that evoked by brushing when the conditioning stimulation was applied at C fiber strength. Note also that the evoked activity in the motor axons was inhibited more by conditioning stimulation than that in the dorsal horn cells in general. (Modified from [54])

Analgesic Effect Tested Using Pain Responses to Natural Stimuli

The experimental animal models described above seem to be useful for studying peripheral conditioning stimulation produced analgesia. However, these models are based primarily on the inhibitory effect of peripheral nerve conditioning stimulation on electrically-evoked responses to peripheral nerve stimulation. Therefore, it is not absolutely certain that the elicited responses are "pain responses" and that the effects produced by peripheral conditioning stimulation are "analgesic effects". A study was recently conducted to test the effects of conditioning stimulation of a peripheral nerve on the activity of dorsal horn cells evoked by natural forms of stimuli applied to the receptive fields in the unanesthetized, decerebrate/ spinal cat [16, 54]. The responses of spinal neurons were evoked by noxious and innocuous mechanical stimuli. Conditioning stimulation of a peripheral nerve produced a powerful inhibition of the responses elicited by noxious stimuli, suggesting that this inhibition is an analgesic effect. Furthermore, the inhibition was differentially greater on the responses to noxious than to innocuous stimuli as shown in Fig. 7. Selective reduction of nociceptive responses of dorsal horn cells were observed earlier by Pomeranz and Cheng [57].

149

Sensitivity Difference Between Analgesic Tests

Indices commonly used to determine levels of pain in experimental animals include measurement of various types of behavioral signs (e.g., vocalization), autonomic motor reactions (e.g., pupil size, blood pressure), somatic motor reactions (e.g., flexion reflex), and activity of nociceptive tract neurons (e.g., dorsal horn cells, STT cells). My tests mainly depend on two of the above indices, the flexion reflex and the activity of nociceptive tract neurons. In an attempt to determine the sensitivity for detecting analgesic effects between two tests, a study was conducted to compare the effects of conditioning stimulation of a peripheral nerve on the activity of dorsal horn neurons and motor axons evoked by noxious stimuli applied to the receptive fields [16, 54]. Comparison was also made of activities evoked by noxious mechanical and thermal stimuli. The reflex activity recorded in motor axons was found to be more sensitive than the activity of dorsal horn cells. The magnitude of the analgesic effect was bigger for the responses to noxious thermal than to mechanical stimuli (Fig. 7). Therefore, among the combination of methods tested, the most sensitive one for detecting analgesic effects produced by conditioning stimulation of a peripheral nerve seems to be the recording of reflex activity of motor neurons elicited by noxious thermal stimuli. Perhaps because of this high sensitivity, many analgesic effects have been successfully demonstrated using the tail flick test [19, 33, 60, 75], a form of reflex motor activity elicited by noxious thermal stimuli.

Problems Associated with Acupuncture Research

Acupuncture is methodologically defined as a procedure, and yet there is no standard procedure. Traditional acupuncture can be defined as a procedure that involves the insertion of acupuncture needles into acupuncture points and the application of mechanical stimulation by manually rotating and moving the needles in and out to treat a disease or to relieve the symptoms of a disease. A number of questions arise from this definition. Is a procedure that applies the same stimulation with a nonacupuncture needle still acupuncture? Is a procedure that applies the same stimulation into nonacupuncture points still acupuncture?

The problem is much worse in electroacupuncture. Electroacupuncture is a procedure that stimulates acupuncture points electrically by passing current through acupuncture needles inserted into the points. If one applies the electrical stimulation through hypodermic needles instead of acupuncture needles, is this procedure electroacupuncture? What should the parameters (intensity, frequency, and patterns) of electrical stimulation be to qualify as electroacupuncture? How deeply do the electrodes have to be inserted into the tissue? Can stimulation through a surface electrode be called electroacupuncture? What would then be the critical difference between electroacupuncture and TENS?

There have been some attempts to define acupuncture effects. One notable example is a proposal made by Andersson [1], when comparing the effects of TENS and acupuncture. He proposed that acupuncture be defined as needle manipulation producing the "De Qi" sensation and electrical stimulation at low frequencies (below 10 Hz) given at an intensity producing more than local muscle contractions. TENS was proposed to be defined as stimulation at higher frequencies. According to Andersson [1], TENS produces a rapidly developing, short lasting, and segmentally distributed analgesia, whereas acupuncture results in an analgesia that has a slow onset, is long lasting, and may be nonsegmentally distributed. However, there are a number of exceptions to this in published results, as reviewed elsewhere [15]. For example, TENS with high frequency (70-200 Hz) reportedly resulted in analgesia lasting longer than 2 h [9, 47]. Pertovaara et al. [55] reported that stimulation with bursts of pulses repeated at 2.5 Hz produced analgesia that could be observed only during stimulation.

Since acupuncture is a methodologically defined term, acupuncture applied with different methods may produce analgesia through different mechanisms. It is most likely that peripheral nerve stimulation produces analgesia through multiple mechanisms. A particular method of stimulation may favor one mechanism, whereas other methods may elicit other mechanisms. Therefore, it is very important to review the published literature while keeping in mind the particular method employed for each study. Part of the confusion in the acupuncture literature may be due to the production of analgesia through different mechanisms in different studies, depending on the methods employed. For example, frequently cited literature for the central structures involved in acupuncture analgesia include studies by Du et al. [20] and Shen et al. [64]. These studies observed a fast onset, short lasting, inhibitory effect of a viscero-somatic reflex by electroacupuncture at high frequency (25-100 Hz). The results of these studies may not apply to acupuncture effects produced at low frequency (2-4 Hz) since the mere act of acupuncture does not necessarily produce an analgesic effect by the same mechanism that underlies typical acupuncture effects.

Summary

This is a brief review of attempts to investigate the peripheral and spinal mechanisms underlying acupuncture analgesia. The basic approach has been the electrophysiological recording of neuronal activity from the spinal cord, which can be used as a nociceptive index, and its modulation by electrical stimulation of a peripheral nerve in experimental animals. Two experimental animal models have been developed. In one, the late component of the flexion reflex in spinal cats was used as a nociceptive index. In the other, activity of STT cells in monkeys evoked by unmyelinated fibers in a peripheral nerve was used as a nociceptive index. In both models, prolonged repetitive stimulation of a peripheral nerve was shown to produce an antinociceptive effect which is largely dependent on spinal mechanisms. The analgesic effect produced consists of two components, naloxone reversible and non-naloxone reversible. The non-naloxone-reversible component is very powerful and develops quickly, but it lasts only a short period, whereas the naloxone-reversible component is less powerful, develops slowly and lasts a long time. My effort has been concentrated mainly on the non-naloxone-reversible component of the antinociceptive effect because I was attracted by its powerful effect. The most important afferent fibers responsible for the antinociceptive effect were found to be in the $A\delta$ group. Within the range tested (0.5–20 Hz), higher frequencies of stimulation were more effective in producing the antinociceptive effect than lower frequencies. The inhibition produced by peripheral conditioning stimulation was differentially greater on the responses to noxious than to innocuous stimuli. The magnitude of the antinociceptive effect is larger for the responses to noxious thermal than to mechanical stimuli. Furthermore, the reflex activity recorded in motor axons seems to be more sensitive than the response of dorsal horn cells.

Finally, lack of a precise and widely accepted definition of "acupuncture" and "acupuncture effect" has been pointed out and is discussed as a problem in the study of acupuncture mechanisms.

Acknowledgments. This work was supported by National Institutes of Health grants NS 21266, NS 11255, and Research Career Development Award NS 00995 to J.M.Chung. The author thanks Heidi Freeborn for the art work and photography.

References

1. Andersson SA (1979) Pain control by sensory stimulation. In: Bonica JJ, Liebeskind JC, Albe-Fessard DG (eds) Advances in pain research and therapy, vol 3. Raven, New York, pp 569–585
2. Andersson SA, Ericson T, Holmgren E, Lindqvist G (1973) Electroacupuncture. Effect on pain threshold measured with electrical stimulation of teeth. Brain 63: 393–396
3. Chang H (1979) Acupuncture analgesia today. Chin Med J [Engl] 92: 7–16
4. Chapman CR, Benedetti C, Colpitts YH, Gerlach R (1983) Naloxone fails to reverse pain thresholds elevated by acupuncture: acupuncture analgesia reconsidered. Pain 16: 13–31
5. Chen G (1980) Acupuncture anesthesia in neurosurgery. Am J Chin Med 8: 271–282
6. Chen GS, Hwang YC (1977) Therapeutic effect of acupuncture for chronic pain. Am J Chin Med 5: 45–61
7. Chen L, Tang J, Fang X, Wang K, Yan JQ (1979) A study of the afferent fibres for the impulses of acupuncture analgesia. National symposium of acupuncture and moxibustion and acupuncture anaesthesia. Beijing, June 1–5, 1979, pp 406–407
8. Cheng C, Ma C, Hsu Y (1979) The groups of afferent fibres responsible for the inhibition induced by electric acupuncture at "neiguan" point. Natl Symposia Acupuncture & Moxibustion & Acupuncture Anaesthesia. pp 407–408, Beijing, June 1–5, 1979
9. Cheng RSS, Pomeranz B (1979) Electroacupuncture analgesia could be mediated by at least two pain-relieving mechanisms; endorphin and non-endorphin systems. Life Sci 25: 1957–1962
10. Cheng SB, Ding LK (1973) Practical application of acupuncture analgesia. Nature 242: 559–560
11. Chiang C, Chang C, Chu H, Yang L (1973) Peripheral afferent pathway for acupuncture analgesia. Sci Sin [B] 16: 210–217
12. Chung JM, Fang ZR, Cargill CL, Willis WD (1983) Prolonged, naloxone-reversible inhibition of the flexion reflex in the cat. Pain 15: 35–53
13. Chung JM, Fang ZR, Hori Y, Lee KH, Willis WD (1984a) Prolonged inhibition of primate spinothalamic tract cells by peripheral nerve stimulation. Pain 19: 259–275
14. Chung JM, Kenshalo DR, Gerhart KD, Willis WD (1979) Excitation of primate spinothalamic neurons by cutaneous C-fiber volleys. J Neurophysiol 42: 1354–1369
15. Chung JM, Lee KH, Hori Y, Endo K, Willis WD (1984b) Factors influencing peripheral nerve stimulation produced inhibition of primate spinothalamic tract cells. Pain 19: 277–293

16. Chung JM, Paik KS, Nam SC (1987) Peripheral conditioning stimulation produces differentially greater antinociceptive effect on noxious thermal response in the cat. Pain, [Suppl 4] S 354, Vth world congress on pain, Hamburg, August 2-7, 1987

17. Chung JM, Paik KS, Nam TS, Kim IK, Kang DH (1981) Morphine sensitive components of the flexion reflex. J Korean Physiol 15: 1-6

18. Croze S, Antonietti C, Duclaux R (1976) Changes in burning pain threshold induced by acupuncture in man. Brain Res 104: 335-340

19. D'Amour FE, Smith DL (1941) A method for determining loss of pain sensation. J Pharmacol Exp Ther 72: 74-79

20. Du H, Chai Y (1976) Localization of central structures involved in descending inhibitory effect of acupuncture on viscero-somatic reflex discharges. Sci Sin [B] 19: 137-148

21. Eriksson MBE, Sjolund BH, Nielzen S (1979) Long term results of peripheral conditioning stimulation as an analgesic measure in chronic pain. Pain 6: 335-347

22. Fleck H (1975) Acupuncture and neurophysiology. Bull NY Acad Med 51: 903-913

23. Foreman RD, Schmidt RF, Willis WD (1979) Effects of mechanical and chemical stimulation of fine muscle afferents upon primate spinothalamic tract cells. J Physiol (Lond) 286: 215-231

24. Fox EJ, Melzack R (1976) Transcutaneous electrical stimulation and acupuncture: comparison of treatment for low-back pain. Pain 2: 141-148

25. Funakoshi M, Kawakita K (1980) Neurophysiological demonstration of an acupuncture point in man. Am J Chin Med 8: 367-369

26. Fung DTH, Hwang JC, Chan SHH, Chin YC (1975) Electro-acupuncture suppression of jaw depression reflex elicited by dentalgia in rabbits. Exp Neurol 47: 367-369

27. Gerhart KD, Wilcox TK, Chung JM, Willis WD (1981) Inhibition of nociceptive and nonnociceptive responses of primate spinothalamic cells by stimulation in medial brainstem. J Neurophysiol 45: 121-136

28. Haber LH, Martin RF, Chung JM, Willis WD (1980) Inhibition and excitation of primate spinothalamic tract neurons by stimulation in region of nucleus reticularis gigantocellularis. J Neurophysiol 43: 1578-1593

29. Han YP, Lee HJ, Chung JM, Paik KS, Nam TS (1980) Experimental study for the central reflex are of the flexion reflex. Yonsei Med J 13: 231-242

29a. Han JS, Terenius L (1982) Neurochemical basis of acupuncture analgesia. Ann Rev Pharmacol Toxicol 22: 193-220

30. Hayes RL, Price DD, Ruda M, Dubner R (1979) Suppression of nociceptive responses in the primate by electrical stimulation of the brain or morphine administration: behavioral and electrophysiological comparisons. Brain Res 167: 417-421

31. Hiedl P, Struppler A, Gessler M (1979) Local analgesia by percutaneous electrical stimulation of sensory nerves. Pain 7: 129-134

32. Hollinger I, Richter JA, Pongratz W, Baum M (1979) Acupuncture anesthesia for open heart surgery: a report of 800 cases. Am J Chin Med 7: 77-90

33. Irwin S, Houde RW, Bennett DR, Hendershot LC, Seevers MH (1951) The effects of morphine, methadone and meperidine on some reflex responses of spinal animals to nociceptive stimulation. J Pharmacol Exp Ther 101: 132-143

34. Jeans ME (1979) Relief of chronic pain by brief, intense transcutaneous electrical stimulation - a double-blind study. In: Bonica JJ (ed) Advances in pain research and therapy. Raven, New York, pp 601-606

35. Kaada B (1974) Mechanisms of acupuncture analgesia. Tidsskr Nor Laegeforen 94: 422-431

36. Kaada B, Hoel E, Leseth K, Nygaard-Ostby B, Setekleiv J, Stovner J (1974) Acupuncture analgesia in the People's Republic of China - with glimpses of other aspects of Chinese medicine. Tidsskr Nor Laegeforen 94: 417-442

37. Kenshalo DR, Leonard RB, Chung JM, Willis WD (1979) Responses of primate spinothalamic neurons to graded and to repeated noxious heat stimuli. J Neurophysiol 42: 1370-1389

38. Kerr FWL, Wilson PR, Nijensohn DE (1978) Acupuncture reduces the trigeminal evoked response in decerebrate cats. Exp Neurol 61: 84-95

39. Kriz N, Sykova E, Vyklicky L (1975) Extracellular potassium changes in the spinal cord of the cat and their relation to slow potentials, active transport and impulse transmission. J Physiol (Lond) 249: 167-182

40. Kuru M (1949) Sensory paths in the spinal cord and brain stem of man. Sogensya, Tokyo

41. Lee KH, Chung JM, Willis WD (1985) Inhibition of primate spinothalamic tract cells by TENS. J Neurosurg 62: 276–287
42. Leung PC (1979) Treatment of low back pain with acupuncture. Am J Chin Med 7: 372–378
43. Levy B, Matsumoto T (1975) Pathophysiology of acupuncture: nervous system transmission. Am Surg 4: 378–384
44. Long DM, Hagfors N (1975) Electrical stimulation in the nervous system: the current status of electrical stimulation of the nervous system for relief of pain. Pain 1: 109–123
45. Lu G, Liang R, Xie J, Wang Y, He G (1979) The role of peripheral nerve fibers in acupuncture analgesia elicited by needling point "zusanli": a physiological analysis. National symposia of acupuncture and moxibustion and acupuncture anesthesia. Beijing, June 1–5, 1979, pp 408–409
46. Lynn B, Perl ER (1977) Failure of acupuncture to produce localized analgesia. Pain 3: 339–351
47. Mannheimer C, Carlsson CA (1979) The analgesic effect of transcutaneous electrical nerve stimulation (TENS) in patients with rheumatoid arthritis. A comparative study of different pulse patterns. Pain 6: 329–334
48. Matsumoto T, Ambruso V, Levy BA, Bednanek J (1974) Acupuncture analgesia in animals: study of specific location(s) of acupuncture points. Am Surg 40: 340–344
49. Mayer DJ, Price DD, Rafii A (1977) Antagonism of acupuncture analgesia in man by the narcotic antagonist naloxone. Brain Res 121: 368–372
50. Melzack R (1975) Prolonged relief of pain by brief, intense transcutaneous somatic stimulation. Pain 1: 357–373
51. Nam SC, Paik KS, Chung JM (1987) Effects of sodium pentobarbital on the activity of different classes of spinal neurons. Neurosci Abstr (In press)
52. Noordenbos W, Wall PD (1976) Diverse sensory functions with an almost totally divided spinal cord. A case of spinal cord transection with preservation of part of one anterolateral quadrant. Pain 2: 185–195
53. Paik KS, Chung JM, Nam TS, Kang DH (1981) Effect of electrical stimulation of peripheral nerve on pain reaction. Korean J Physiol 15: 7–17
54. Paik KS, Nam SC, Chung JM (1988) Differential inhibition produced by peripheral conditioning stimulation on noxious mechanical and thermal responses of different classes of spinal neurons in the cat. Exp Neurol 99: 498–511
55. Pertovaara A, Kemppainen P, Johansson G, Karonen SL (1982) Dental analgesia produced by non-painful, low-frequency stimulation is not influenced by stress or reversed by naloxone. Pain 13: 379–384
56. Picaza JA, Cannon BW, Hunter SE, Boyd AS, Guma J, Maurer D (1975) Pain suppression by peripheral nerve stimulation. Part I. Observations with transcutaneous stimuli. Surg Neurol 4: 105–114
57. Pomeranz B, Cheng R (1979) Suppression of noxious responses in single neurons of cat spinal cord by electroacupuncture and its reversal by the opiate antagonist naloxone. Exp Neurol 64: 327–341
58. Pomeranz B, Chiu D (1976) Naloxone blockade of acupuncture analgesia: endorphin implicated. Life Sci 19: 1757–1762
59. Pomeranz B, Paley D (1979) Electroacupuncture hypalgesia is mediated by afferent nerve impulses: an electrophysiological study in mice. Exp Neurol 66: 398–402
60. Sandkuhler J, Gebhart GF (1984) Characterization of inhibition of a spinal nociceptive reflex by stimulation medially and laterally in the midbrain and medulla in the pentobarbital-anesthetized rat. Brain Res 305: 67–76
61. Sechzer PH, Leung SJ (1975) Acupuncture: surgical aspects. Bull NY Acad Med 51: 922–929
62. Shanghai Acupuncture Anesthesia Coordinating Group (1975) Acupuncture anesthesia. An anesthetic method combining traditional Chinese and Western medicine. Chin Med J [Engl] 1: 13–27
63. Shealy CN (1974) Transcutaneous electrical stimulation for control of pain. Clin Neurosurg 21: 269–277
64. Shen E, Ts'ai T, Lan C (1975) Supraspinal participation in the inhibitory effect of acupuncture on viscero-somatic reflex discharges. Chin Med J [Engl] 1: 431–440

154

65. Sherrington CS (1910) Flexion-reflex of the limb, crossed extension reflex, and reflex stepping and standing. J Physiol 40: 28-121
66. Shin HK, Kim J, Chung JM (1986) Inhibition and excitation of the nociceptive flexion reflex by conditioning stimulation of a peripheral nerve in the cat. Exp Neurol 92: 335-348
67. Sjolund BH, Eriksson MBE (1979) The influence of naloxone on analgesia produced by peripheral conditioning stimulation. Brain Res 173: 295-301
68. Sjolund BH, Eriksson MBE (1976) Electro-acupuncture and endogenous morphines. Lancet 2: 1085
69. Toda K, Ichioka M (1978) Electroacupuncture: relations between forelimb afferent impulses and suppression of jaw-opening reflex in the rat. Exp Neurol 61: 465-470
70. Van Nghi N (1973) Acupuncture anesthesia. Am J Chin Med 1: 135-142
71. Vierck CJ, Luck MM (1979) Loss and recovery of reactivity to noxious stimuli in monkeys with primary spinothalamic cordotomies, followed by secondary and tertiary lesions of other cord sectors. Brain 102: 233-248
72. White JC, Sweet WH (1955) Pain, its mechanisms and neurosurgical control. Thomas, Springfield
73. Woolf CJ (1979) Transcutaneous electrical nerve stimulation and the reaction to experimental pain in human subjects. Pain 7: 115-127
74. Woolf CJ, Mitchell D, Barrett GD (1980) Antinociceptive effect of peripheral segmental electrical stimulation in the rat. Pain 8: 237-252
75. Yeung JC, Yakash TL, Rudy TA (1977) Current mapping of brain sites for sensitivity to the direct application of morphine and focal electrical stimulation in the production of antinociception in the rat. Pain 4: 23-40

Clinical and Research Observations on Acupuncture Analgesia and Thermography

Mathew H. M. Lee[1] and Monique Ernst[2]

[1] New York University, Goldwater Memorial Hospital, Franklin D. Roosevelt Island, New York, N.Y. 10044, USA
[2] Chronic Pain Unit, Goldwater Memorial Hospital, New York University Medical Center, and Department of Psychiatry, Beth Israel Medical Center, New York, N.Y. 10044, USA

Introduction

The concept of acupuncture become popular among the American medical community and lay public as a potential therapeutic tool following the American rapprochement with the People's Republic of China in 1972. They found this idea both exciting and vaguely unsettling to their accustomed ways of thinking.

I (Lee) was privileged to be selected to accompany a group of Chinese-American medical scholars to visit the People's Republic of China upon the invitation of Chairman Mao. During the 7-week visit in 1973, various surgical, dental, and medical acupuncture procedures were observed. I visited various researchers, especially Dr. Chang Hsiang-Tung at the Shanghai Scientific Institute of Physiology.

In 1973, New York State established a Commission on Acupuncture to promote scientific inquiry and appropriate training of practitioners, and to protect the public from harm and exploitation. Having been named to this Commission commenced my initial reluctant journey into an exciting area of pursuit.

It became obvious that the patient with chronic pain that could be safely helped with acupuncture was in no mood to wait for research results. The resolution of this paradox was self-evident: We needed to make clinical observations first and then return to the laboratories. The challenge presented by such a research effort was heightened by the possibilities for uncovering basic neurological, biophysical, and biochemical knowledge about the functioning of the human body that heretofore had remained unknown. In addition, the prospect of adding acupuncture to the armamentarium of pain therapy and dental analgesia appeared to be an exciting challenge.

Our initial work involved the observation of acupuncture analgesia in dentistry followed by the development of a precision tooth pulp stimulation technique for assessment of the pain threshold. Subsequently, an acupuncture dental pain research model was born. We then became involved in testing aspirin and other medication to see how they altered these thresholds, as compared with acupuncture. Naloxone was also given. Our focus, in terms of acupuncture stimulation points, was directed at the first dorsal interosseous muscle (LI. 4 Hegu) and the tibialis anterior muscle (St. 36 Zusanli). More recently, we have enlisted thermography to evaluate the sympathetic effects of acupuncture. This chapter will summarize our findings.

Clinical Dental Analgesia

Based on observations in the People's Republic of China, we decided to attempt first to investigate the use of acupuncture clinically for inducing analgesia in routine dental procedures. The major purposes of this investigation were to attempt to replicate findings reported in the Chinese literature and to assess the feasibility of acupuncture analgesia as an alternative method for achieving anesthesia in treating dental problems.

Methodology

Twenty subjects, ten males and ten females, volunteered for participation in this study [37a]. All subjects were between 18 and 30 years of age, in good health, and were in need of routine dental treatment. All subjects had a history of previous dental care with local anesthetic.

Prior to undergoing any treatment, all subjects were interviewed to determine their attitudes toward dental treatment and to obtain some background on their knowledge and impressions of acupuncture. Immediately after this brief interview, the subjects were brought to a dental treatment area where they were seated in the dental chair and the acupuncture procedure initiated. Sterilized standard steel 27-gauge needles were used for the acupuncture procedure. Prior to insertion of the needles, the selected areas on the skin were swabbed with alcohol sponges. Analgesia was attempted by the induction of acupuncture needles at the two LI.4 Hegu points and at the ipsilateral temporal mandibular joint area. In order to achieve and maintain any analgesic effect, the needles were continuously manipulated throughout the dental procedure. At brief intervals, testing was conducted to determine whether an acceptable analgesic effect had been achieved. Such testing involved applying pressure with a dental explorer to the gingival tissues of the area to be treated or piercing the mucous membranes in the problem area with the point of the explorer. Only when complete analgesia was obtained was any dental treatment initiated. Continuous monitoring of patient reactions was diligently observed throughout the course of the procedure. To provide additional subjective information during treatment, each subject was encouraged to give verbal reports of his or her reactions, including the occurrence of any sensations or other physiological changes. If analgesia was deemed ineffective at any point during the procedure, then the dental treatment was stopped. Before continuing any further dental work, anesthesia was induced by the conventional method of procaine nerve block.

In no instance was any premedication given to the subjects. At the completion of the dental procedure, each subject was kept under observation for a minimum of 1 h, and all subjects were given scheduled appointments for follow-up observation on the day after treatment. In addition, at the conclusion of the dental procedure, each subject was again interviewed briefly to determine individual reactions to the entire procedure.

Results

Of the 20 cases included in the study, 16 were deemed totally successful: the major criterion was the maintenance of a satisfactory analgesic effect throughout the entire course of the dental procedures performed.

Among the types of dental problems successfully treated with acupuncture, 7 cases were tooth extractions, of which one was an impacted tooth with surgical removal of bone with mallet and chisel as well as motor-driven instrumentation, 12 cases involved cavity preparation and complete removal of caries, and 1 case involved deep gingival scaling and curettage. (Note: these figures are based on the fact that, for several of the subjects, more than one dental procedure was performed.) Of the remaining 4 cases, one was not successful. For the other three, a degree of acupuncture analgesia was obtained, but it could not be adequately maintained to complete the required dental procedure.

Monitoring of each subject during the acupuncture procedure showed that, on average, an analgesic effect could be obtained in about 3 min from insertion of the first needle. Moreover, at the completion of the dental procedure, the subjects reported the return of sensation approximately 30 s after termination of the manipulation of the needles.

In those cases in which acupuncture was successful, the patients reported no side effects during or after treatment, a general positive reaction and willingness to repeat the procedure, and a greater decrease in posttreatment discomfort as compared with standard anesthetic techniques. Postoperative bleeding was minimal and in no case were postoperative analgesics required. Additionally, in each of the cases, there was no evidence of edema or postoperative complications. As a result, most of these subjects preferred acupuncture analgesia to the standard methods of anesthesia usually employed in their previous dental treatments.

Acupuncture Dental Pain Research Model

With an 80% success rate in our dental clinical experience, it was mandatory to reassess our position – thus, the evolution of our acupuncture dental pain research model. What was needed was an accurate, replicable pain stimulus model (Fig. 1). Obviously the tooth, innervated by sensory fibers only, appeared ideal. A new technique for administering electrical stimulation to the dental pulp provided a precise, well-quantified measurement for assessing the efficacy of a variety of analgesic agents [14]. The test was developed in collaboration with Dr. Barry Dworkin, Rockefeller University. Its reliability and validity for measuring pain intensity were established in double-blind pharmacological studies, using aspirin, codeine, and placebo [39]. The dental stimulation technique optimized accuracy, reliability, and comfort for the subject [14] and permitted repeated pain measurements during prolonged sessions as well as at intervals of months without any change in the baseline condition. Special consideration was given to insure constancy of the current density delivered to the pulp nerve as well as to free the subject from holding the stimulation device in place. The use of a therapeutic filling as the cathode provided a constant geometrical relationship between the pulp

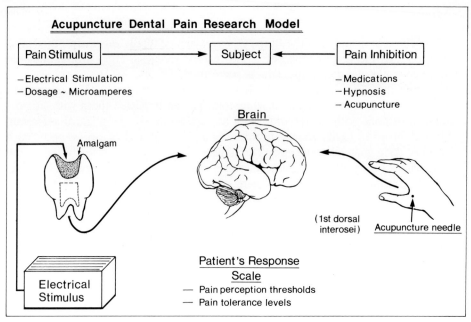

Fig. 1. Acupuncture dental pain research model

nerve and the electrode of stimulation (Fig. 2). The fabrication of an individual rubber mold containing the electrode of stimulation (platinum EEG Grass electrode), by preventing saliva leak, and by its watertight adhesion to the stimulated region, maintained the resistance of the preparation constant (Fig. 3). This technique was designed for cross-over experiments. The use of well-trained subjects minimized stress factors.

We examined, in humans, the analgesic effects of nonsegmental electroacupuncture (EA) limited to a single point LI. 4 Hegu and the influence of naloxone on experimental pain [16].

Electroacupuncture analgesia is well documented in the clinical pain [11, 20, 41, 55] as well as in experimental pain literature [9, 27, 44, 51]. Numerous studies have implicated the endogenous opioid system in its mechanism of action [24, 56, 58]. However this subject is still controversial, especially with regard to the effect of naloxone, a specific narcotic antagonist agent [54], on the analgesic effect [8, 44, 49]. Many factors account for the discrepancy in the results of the naloxone studies, including the type of experimental pain model.

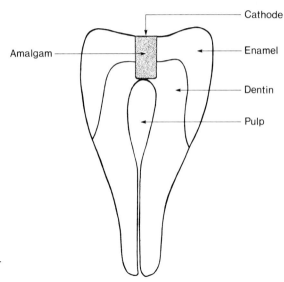

Fig.2. Sagittal view of the tooth. The dental filling is used as the electrode of stimulation

Methods

Five normal female paid subjects (25–35 years old) participated in 65 sessions under four conditions (control, EA, EA+naloxone, EA+placebo). Each subject was fully accustomed to the experimental procedure at the beginning of the experiment, after having participated in preliminary training sessions. The sessions were 60 min long and consisted of seven pain measurements at 10-minute intervals. They were performed at the same time of day, at 1-week intervals. Session order was randomized.

The pain measurement consisted of the evaluation of two pain levels: pain detection determined by the lowest intensity of stimulation consistently perceived by the subject, and pain discomfort determined by the intensity of stimulation which, if persisting, would prompt the subject to take a pain relief agent.

Experimental dental pain was produced by electrical stimulation (600-ms train of 100×1 ms rectangular pulses, intensity range between 0 and 500 µA) delivered by a constant current stimulator to a therapeutic filling of a molar or premolar of the superior jaw. This technique has been described in detail previously [14]. The electrode of stimulation (EEG Grass Instrument) was inserted into a silicone rubber mold which isolated the filling from the saliva and the buccal mucosa. The indifferent electrode, composed of three gold disk electrodes, was placed in the buccal pouch. Pain thresholds were determined through the method of ascending limits [65] for which stimuli were delivered every 8 s.

The electroacupuncture (EA) was delivered to the right Hegu hand point with a sterile Chinese acupuncture needle. The LI.4 Hegu point, located in the first dorsal interosseus muscle, has been used extensively in acupuncture studies due to its well-known orofacial analgesic effects [2, 61]. The electrical stimulation consisted of a 0.8-ms rectangular pulse delivered at 2-Hz frequency by a constant current stimulator. The intensity was adjusted to a level slightly above pain threshold,

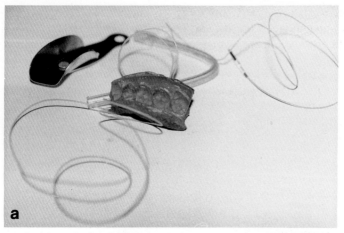

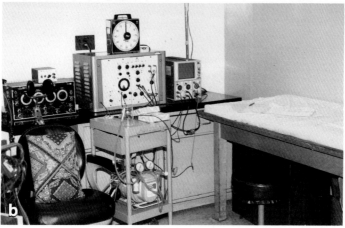

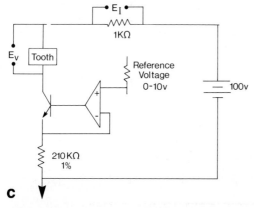

Fig. 3. a Silicone rubber mold showing electrode and Teflon-insulated connecting wire. **b** Experimental setting. The subject signals perception of the stimulus by pressing a button on either side which lights the experimenter's panel. **c** A partial schematic diagram of the current control section of the stimulator. Note that the reference ground is isolated. E_I and E_V are used to calculate the preparation impedance

which provoked muscular twitches (8-15 mA). EA was initiated after the first pain measurement and was maintained until the end of the session. Although unpleasant, the EA stimulation was reported to be quite bearable and not disturbing to concentration.

In the pharmacological sessions, a brachial biceps intramuscular injection of either 0.8 mg naloxone (4 cc) or isotonic saline (4 cc) was given after the second pain measurement in a double-blind procedure.

The results were analyzed by means of a three-way analysis of variance [31].

Results

Dental pain detection and pain discomfort thresholds remained stable during the control condition with a fluctuation range of $2\% \pm 1\%$. In contrast, they increased progressively and significantly ($P < 0.0001$) during EA treatment (27% increase with 60-min EA). The magnitude of the threshold increase at 60 min was similar for the detection level and the discomfort level (detection $27.5\% \pm 3.1\%$, discomfort $27.1\% \pm 2.8$). This increase was partially blocked by the double blind intramuscular injection of 0.8 mg naloxone ($P < 0.005$) (Figs. 4, 5). The experimental

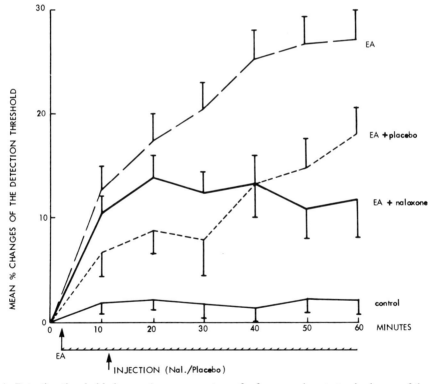

Fig. 4. Detection threshold changes (mean percentage of reference values ± standard error of the mean) during 60-min period under four conditions: *control* ($n = 18$), *EA* ($n = 22$), *EA + naloxone* ($n = 14$), and *EA + placebo* ($n = 11$) in five subjects

163

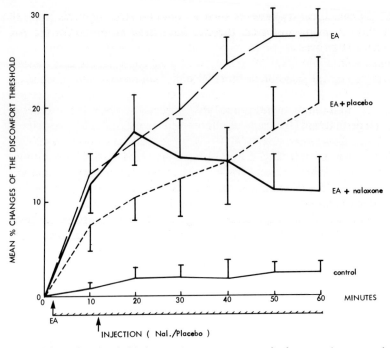

Fig. 5. Discomfort threshold changes (mean percentage of reference values ± standard error of the mean) during 60-min period under four conditions: *control* ($n = 18$), *EA* ($n = 22$), *EA + naloxone* ($n = 14$), and *EA + placebo* ($n = 11$) in five subjects

conditions were carefully controlled in order to prevent the occurrence of a stress analgesic effect.

Discussion

The absence of a differential analgesic effect of acupuncture on low and high pain sensory levels is in contrast with the findings of Chapman et al. (1976) who reported a stronger acupuncture effect on low pain intensity than on high pain intensity [10]. The use of pain discomfort threshold rather than pain tolerance threshold may account for this discrepancy. However, the degree of pain threshold increase (27%) found in our study is in accordance with the reports in the literature. Mayer et al. (1977) observed a 27% increase of dental pain thresholds after 30 min of LI.4 Hegu manual acupuncture [44]. Lynn et al. (1977) reported a 20% pain relief in patients after nonsegmental EA [42]. A review of the literature indicates that segmental EA yields a stronger pain threshold increase: 40% reported by Sjolund et al. (1979) [57], 57% reported by Fox et al. (1976) [20], and 87% reported by Chapman et al. (1977) [9]. This discrepancy suggests that segmental acupuncture activates more efficiently than nonsegmental acupuncture a central analgesic system, or that it triggers an additional specific segmental analgesic system.

164

Apart from psychological hypotheses such as placebo [46], hypnosis [29, 33], and stress [8], three neurophysiological theories have been proposed for the EA analgesic mechanism of action.

1. A segmental spinal inhibition of nociceptive inputs based on the gate control theory [45] results in an immediate, short-lasting, segmental, and nonopioid analgesia.

2. The central, endogenous, opioid, analgesic system accounts for a general, long-lasting, analgesic effect [43].

3. The third hypothesis involves the activation of the diffuse noxious inhibitory controls (DNIC), recently introduced by LeBars et al. (1981) [34]. These authors reported the spinal inhibition of convergent cells of the dorsal horn by nonsegmental peripheral noxious stimulations in rats. Nonconvergent cells were not affected, and nonnoxious stimulations were ineffective.

The partial blockade of the acupuncture analgesic effect by naloxone suggests the implication of endogenous opioid substances in EA analgesia. It does not support the hypothesis of psychological factors as the unique basis for acupuncture analgesia. Indeed, most studies agree on the absence of naloxone influence at low dosage (<2 mg) on the analgesia produced by either placebo [40] or by hypnosis [23, 47, 60]. The naloxone-insensitive component of EA analgesia may be accounted for by psychological factors as well as by non-opioid neurophysiological analgesic systems. In addition, there has recently been a growing interest in the study of the relationship between the sympathetic nervous system and pain modulation [17, 18]. Edwall et al. (1971) [15] suggested that the pulp nerve activity is modulated by the local vasomotor tone, which in turn may be modified by EA treatment.

In conclusion, this study is evidence of the analgesic effect of nonsegmental EA of a single point on experimental dental pain and its partial reversal by naloxone 0.8 mg IM. This finding suggests that the endogenous opioid system is activated either by a specific acupuncture mechanism, or by a nonspecific one such as the DNIC system or the sympathetic nervous system.

The Sympathetic Effect of Acupuncture

The studies which have attempted to appraise the role of the sympathetic nervous system in acupuncture show contradictory findings. Some authors report an increase in the sympathetic activity following acupuncture upon the cardiovascular function in dogs [35]. Others report a decrease in the sympathetic tone resulting in peripheral vasodilation [36, 38]. Omura [50] reports a transient increase followed by a long-lasting decrease in the sympathetic activity. The discrepancy in the findings stems from the difficulty in monitoring sympathetic activity, as well as from the different types of acupuncture techniques. The recent use of thermography [5] in the medical field represents a major advance for clinical research by providing a simple, reliable, and sensitive tool for assessing peripheral sympathetic activity through measurements of surface skin temperature.

We conducted experiments to assess the peripheral sympathetic effect of manual and electrical acupuncture, as well as the central autonomic effect of manual acupuncture, by means of, respectively, thermography and cardiorespiratory function measurements (blood pressure, heart rate, and respiratory quotient).

Thermography Studies: Measurement of Peripheral Sympathetic Activity

Skin temperature is a function of blood perfusion, which represents an index of sympathetic activity. The increase in sympathetic vasomotor tone induces vasoconstriction and hence decreases skin temperature. Conversely, the decrease in sympathetic vasomotor tone induces vasodilation and thus increases skin temperature. Thermographic scans visualize surface temperature and, by recording all body temperature, permit the differentiation of regional, segmental, and central sympathetic changes. In a preliminary report [37] we demonstrated via thermography a skin temperature (Tsk) rise in both hands of three subjects after unilateral LI.4 Hegu manual acupuncture, which suggested a sympatholytic effect. This finding gave rise to two experiments measuring skin temperature changes in the face, hands, and feet after manual acupuncture and electrical acupuncture of the LI.4 Hegu hand point in the first experiment [17], and of the St.36 Zusanli knee point in the second experiment [18]. Both acupuncture modalities (electrical and manual) were used since there is evidence of a specific analgesic response pattern according to the type of acupuncture technique. Generalized analgesia is described with manual acupuncture [3, 12, 48] and segmental analgesia with electrical stimulation [45, 63].

Methods

Nineteen normal subjects (32 ± 8 years old; 17 females and 2 males) were used in both experiments which were performed at 3-week intervals. The sessions, control, manual acupuncture (MA), and EA, were randomly distributed. The subjects were instructed not to eat, drink, or smoke at least 2 h prior to the session. The experimental room was at a constant temperature of 23 °C and draft free. A 20-min rest period at the start of each session acclimatised the subject to the experimental setting and stabilized Tsk.

Temperature of the hands, feet, and face were recorded by means of an infrared color thermograph (Inframetrics, Model 525). Each session lasted about 1 h. Basal Tsk was recorded at t_0, immediately after the rest period. Color slides of the thermograms of the hand dorsum, foot dorsum, and face were taken every 5 min during the following 30 min.

In the acupuncture sessions, a sterile Chinese acupuncture needle was inserted in the left LI.4 Hegu point (first dorsal interosseus muscle) or in the left St.36 Zusanli point (motor point of the tibialis anterior muscle) [2] immediately after the first temperature recording and was removed 15 min later (t_{15}). Temperature recording was continued for another 15-min period (t_{30}). MA consisted of twirling the needle in between temperature recordings, until the subject experienced a painful sensation. EA was delivered to the acupuncture needle by a constant current stimulator. Rectangular 0.8-ms pulses at 1 Hz frequency were adjusted at an

166

pulse shape
pulse width
Hz
Current - mA

intensity strong enough to evoke muscle twitching and sensation of tapping or pounding just below the pain sensation threshold (7-15 mA).

In the control sessions, the subjects were sitting quietly during the whole period of temperature recordings (30 min).

Data was collected by averaging the temperature of standardized areas of each body segment under study.

Left and right hands as well as left and right feet did not show any statistical difference in the Tsk changes. Therefore, they were analyzed as a unit.

A three factor analysis of variance compared the mean Tsk changes at 5 min (t_5), 15 min (t_{15}), and 30 min (t_{30}) after the beginning of the Tsk recording and within the conditions (control, Hegu MA, Hegu EA, Zusanli MA, Zusanli EA). Planned pair-wise comparisons (LSD Fischer test) were made among the means [32]. The criterion for significance was set at $P < 0.05$.

Results

The initial mean Tsk (t_0) of hands, feet, and face was similar in the five conditions. This indicated that the 20-min rest period was adequate to establish homogenous basal Tsk for all five conditions. The analysis of variance showed that all effects and interactions were significant.

MA of both points induced a Tsk increase that was maximal at the end of the session (t_{30}), most significant for the face (F[4,72]=24.26; LSD=0.70; $P < 0.001$), less significant for the hands (F[4,72]=3.07; LSD=2.01; $P < 0.01$), and did not reach the criterion of significance for the feet (F[4,72]=2.77; LSD=1.3; NS). The only statistical difference between the MA effects of both points appeared in the magnitude of the Tsk increase in the face, with the Hegu hand point yielding the strongest effect.

EA of both points induced a Tsk increase in the face, with the LI.4 Hegu hand point yielding the strongest effect. It was maximal at the end of the session and most significant for the face; again the face Tsk increase was significantly greater with LI.4 Hegu point EA than with St.36 Zusanli point EA; in the feet, Hegu point EA increased Tsk, while Zusanli point decreased Tsk (Figs.6, 7).

Compared to the control condition, MA and EA of LI.4 Hegu and St.36 Zusanli points induced a nonsegmental, long-lasting, warming (sympatholytic) effect, which was distributed according to a craniocaudal gradient, i.e., maximum effect in the face, and which was stronger with MA. In addition, EA induced an initial segmental cooling (sympathomimetic) effect (in the hands with LI.4 Hegu point and in the feet with St.36 Zusanli point) that decreased during the remainder of the session.

Discussion

The similar temporal course and spatial distribution of the Tsk changes after stimulation of either a knee point or hand point is consistent with the hypothesis of the activation of a central sympathetic inhibitory system. The somatotopicity of this system is unrelated to the site of peripheral stimulation.

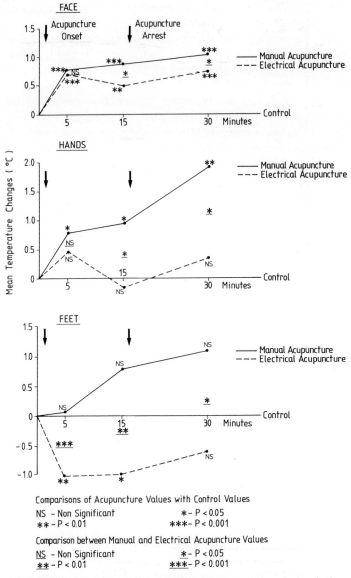

Fig. 6. Mean skin temperature changes during manual and electrical acupuncture of the LI.4 Hegu hand point, with the control values as reference ($n = 19$)

The initial sympathomimetic activation observed after electrical acupuncture reflects the activation of segmental vasomotor reflexes rather than a generalized emotional arousal [6]. This is consistent with Procacci's findings [52] demonstrating a segmental sympathetic reflex by inhibiting skin potential response in both ipsilateral and contralateral limbs, after unilateral sympathetic block. Bilateral connections on a segmental level of the sympathetic innervation are also evi-

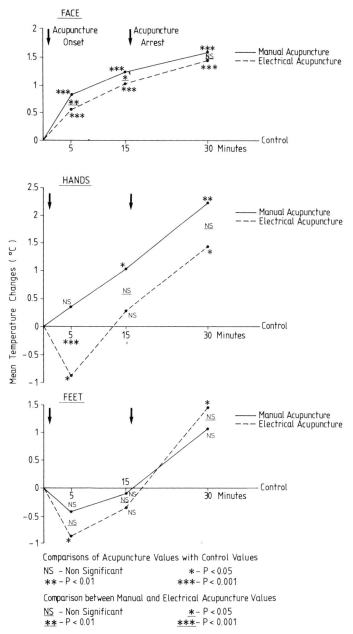

Fig. 7. Mean skin temperature changes during manual and electrical acupuncture of the St. 36 Zusanli knee point, with the control values as reference ($n = 19$)

denced by the well-known "mirror image" of reflex sympathetic dystrophy, which shows a contralateral extension of the dystrophic process. The segmental activation of the sympathetic nervous system is in agreement with the observation of an exacerbation of the sympathetic dystrophy symptoms after transcutaneous electrical stimulation treatment [1]. The short duration of the sympathomimetic effect may result from a depressive effect exerted by the "specific" sympatholytic effect of acupuncture. The development of an adaptation to the repetitive stimulation is unlikely since adaptation of a preganglionic reflex to repetitive stimulation of afferent fibers in the spinal nerves begins at a stimulation frequency of $1/s$ and is complete at rates above $5/s$ [6].

In a larger perspective, although the literature relative to interactions between pain control and the sympathetic nervous system is limited, there is evidence of relationships between both functions. The sympathetic nervous system has been shown to play a significant role in the stabilization of the cutaneous pain threshold in humans [22]. Several analogies between peripheral sympathetic vasomotor tone and pain sensation have been reported: thermography studies identified chronic pain areas as cold spots and acute pain areas as warm spots [19, 62, 64]. Dorsal column stimulation has been associated with a Tsk increase in the region of analgesia [21]. The somatotopically organized analgesic system found in the midbrain area of the rat mirrors the cephalocaudal gradient distribution of the sympatholytic effect observed in our study [53].

Acupuncture analgesia may be mediated at least partly by the central endogenous opioid system [3, 12, 43, 51]. Anatomical, physiological, and pharmacological observations indicate common features of the central endogenous analgesic system and the thermoregulatory function: opiate receptors are found in high concentration in the brain stem and in the hypothalamic thermoregulatory centers [4, 26, 59]. Electrical stimulation of the nucleus raphe magnus has been shown to produce analgesia [48] as well as to inhibit thermogenesis [13]. Serotoninergic systems implicated in acupuncture analgesia [25] are believed to be part of the central thermoregulatory pathway [7]. Administration of morphine and endorphin intravenously and intraventricularly produced hypothermia secondary to peripheral vasodilation and depression of the thermoregulatory center [30, 66]. This strongly suggests that endogenous opioid systems may be involved in the acupuncture sympatholytic effect.

In conclusion, the sympathetic effects of acupuncture found in this study were temporally and spatially similar to two separate acupuncture analgesic mechanisms: (a) the finding of a long-lasting, generalized, sympathetic inhibitory effect with MA correlates with the generalized, endogenous, opioid analgesia produced by MA [3, 12, 43], and (b) the short-term, segmental, sympathetic excitatory effect associated with EA correlates with the segmental spinal analgesia produced by transcutaneous electrical stimulation (TENS) [45, 63].

These sympathetic effects were not observed after TENS (M. Ernst et al., unpublished results). In similar experimental conditions, TENS did not significantly alter skin temperature when compared with sham-TENS. TENS applied to the upper extremity tended to activate peripheral and central sympathetic tone, producing a relative, generalized, cooling effect associated with an increase in heart rate and blood pressure. When applied to the lower extremity, TENS tended to inhibit peripheral and central sympathetic activity, as evidenced by a relative, generalized, warming effect with a decrease in heart rate and diastolic pressure. Kaada reported the occurrence of a widespread and prolonged vasodilation after TENS, which was not influenced by the injection of naloxone but was blocked by the central serotonin blocker cyproheptadine and was accompanied by the peripheral release of an "active" vasodilator [28]. The discrepancy in the results may be accounted for by the differences in the type of TENS techniques and experimental conditions used in both studies. Kaada utilized low-frequency stimulation (2 Hz), similar to the electroacupuncture technique, in patients with vascular disease, with no control group. He recorded skin temperature via a thermistor and an electronic digital thermometer. We used the traditional high-frequency TENS (80 Hz), in normal subjects with a control group, and recorded temperature changes via infrared thermography.

The findings of the above studies suggest differential sympathetic effects of MA, EA, and TENS. Further work is warranted to explore the neurophysiological relationships between the sympathetic and the analgesic effects of acupuncture and TENS.

Central Sympathetic Effects: Effects of Acupuncture on Cardiovascular and Respiratory Function Before, During, and After Exercise

We demonstrated in the above studies the production of peripheral sympathetic effects by acupuncture. We were interested in completing our findings by studying the influence and the modulatory role of acupuncture on central sympathetic activity. We evaluated the effects of MA on cardiorespiratory function under basal (rest) and activation (stress exercise) conditions (M. Ernst et al., unpublished results). We will present only the outlines of this work, which is still in progress.

Methods

Fifteen healthy subjects were randomly assigned to two groups, MA and sham-acupuncture. Each session consisted of 20 min equilibration, 15 min acupuncture/sham, 10 min arm crank exercise, 15 min recovery. Respiratory gas exchange, ECG, and blood pressure were monitored throughout the session under strictly standardized conditions. Manual acupuncture consisted of the bilateral needling of the LI.4 Hegu hand and the St. 36 Zusanli knee points and twirling of the acupuncture needle. Sham-acupuncture consisted of the superficial needling of non-acupuncture points close to the Hegu and Zusanli points and the fake manipulation of the acupuncture needle. Neither the subject nor the experimenter knew the acupuncturist's technique.

Results

In comparison with placebo, acupuncture decreased heart rate ($P < 0.04$) and diastolic pressure ($P < 0.04$) before exercise, and decreased diastolic pressure ($P < 0.05$) and increased respiratory quotient ($P < 0.03$) during and after exercise.

Discussion

Acupuncture produces a sympathetic inhibition, mimicking a beta-blocking effect, dampening the autonomic activation of stress exercise and reducing the cardiac output, which results in a respiratory quotient increase. This is in accordance with previous results showing a generalized decrease of peripheral sympathetic tone after acupuncture [17, 18]. In contrast to the hypothesis of a stress analgesic effect as proposed in the literature for the mechanism of action of acupuncture analgesia [8], this finding does not support the existence of a common sympathetic pathway to acupuncture analgesia and stress analgesia, since acupuncture antagonized stress sympathetic effects.

Future Research Directions

Our laboratory will continue to study the autonomic changes occurring during acupuncture and TENS, using pharmacological challenges, in order to clarify the chemical mediators of these acupuncture effects. The utilization of computerized thermography on a continuous dynamic basis offers a powerful diagnostic tool for the study of pain, acupuncture, and particularly soft tissue damage. We have witnessed that the progression of thermographic changes from a steady resting state to a definitive pain pattern during movement of an extremity correlated with a subject's verbal description.

Our studies clearly indicate that skin surface temperature alteration and patterns following acupuncture therapy can be visualized and measured via thermography. Of course, much delineation and refinement have yet to be resolved.

Therefore, our Chronic Pain Unit plans to direct a major thrust of its research effort into this area and thus hopes to contribute toward elucidating the interactions between sympathetic and analgesic acupuncture effects in clinical and experimental pain.

Summary

After demonstrating an 80% success rate in our dental analgesia studies using acupuncture, we developed an acupuncture dental pain research model utilizing a tooth pulp stimulation technique to measure pain. This technique allowed to measure alterations in pain under various medications, acupuncture and acupuncture challenged by naloxone. The sympathetic effect of acupuncture was observed using thermography as a measurement of peripheral sympathetic activity. A decreased gradient effect was witnessed when the LI.4 Hegu point (as opposed to the St.36 Zusanli point) was stimulated. The central sympathetic effects in terms of acupuncture affecting the cardiovascular and respiratory functions were demonstrated following exercise. Acupuncture produced a sympathetic inhibition mimicking a Beta blocking effect.

References

1. Abram SE (1976) Increased sympathetic tone associated with transcutaneous electrical stimulation. Anesthesiology 45: 575–577
2. Academy of Traditional Chinese Medicine (1975) An outline of chinese acupuncture. Foreign Language Press, Peking, pp 305
3. Akil H, Mayer DJ, Liebeskind JC (1976) Antagonism of stimulation produced analgesia by naloxone, a narcotic antagonist. Science 191: 961–962
4. Atweh SF, Kuhar MJ (1977) Autoradiographic localization of opiate receptors in rat brain: I. Spinal cord and lower medulla. Brain Res 124: 53–67
5. Barnes RB, Gershon-Cohen J (1963) Clinical thermography. JAMA 185: 949–952
6. Beachman WS, Perl ER (1964) Characteristics of a spinal sympathetic reflex. J Physiol (Lond) 173: 431–448
7. Bruck K, Hinckel P (1982) Thermoafferent systems and their adaptive modifications. Pharmacol Ther 17: 357–381
8. Chapman CR, Benedetti C, Colpitis YH, Gerlach R (1983) Naloxone fails to reverse pain thresholds elevated by acupuncture: acupuncture analgesia reconsidered. Pain 16: 13–31
9. Chapman CR, Chen AC, Bonica JJ (1977) Effects of intra-segmental electrical acupuncture on dental pain: evaluation by threshold estimation and sensory decision theory. Pain 3: 213–227
10. Chapman CR, Wilson ME, Gehrig JD (1976) Comparative effects of acupuncture and transcutaneous electrical stimulation of the perception of painful dental stimuli. Pain 2: 265–283
11. Chen GS, Hwang YC, Song SJ (1978) Long-term effect of acupuncture therapy on headache. Am J Acupunct 6: 23–32
12. Cheng RSS, Pomeranz B (1979) Electroacupuncture analgesia could be mediated by at least two pain relieving mechanisms, endorphin and non-endorphin systems. Life Sci 25: 1957–1962
13. Cristante L, Hinckel P, Bruck K (1981) Inhibition of thermogenesis by electrical stimulation of the nucleus raphe magnus. Pflugers Arch 391: 45
14. Dworkin BR, Lee MHM, Zaretsky HH, Berkeley HA (1977) Instrumentation and techniques. A precision tooth-pulp stimulation technique for the assessment of pain. Behav Res Meth Instrum 9: 463–465
15. Edwall L, Scott D (1971) Influence of changes on the excitability of the sensory unit in the tooth of the cat. Acta Physiol Scand 82: 555–556
16. Ernst M, Lee MHM (1987) Influence of naloxone on electroacupuncture analgesia using an experimental dental pain test. Review of possible mechanisms of action. Acupunct Electrother Res 12: 5–22
17. Ernst M, Lee MHM (1986) Sympathetic effects of manual and electrical acupuncture of the Tsusanli knee point: comparison with the Hoku hand point sympathetic effect. Exp Neurol 94: 1–10
18. Ernst M, Lee MHM (1985) Sympathetic vasomotor changes induced by manual and electrical acupuncture of the Hoku point visualized by thermography. Pain 21: 25–33
19. Fischer AA (1981) Thermography and pain. Arch Phys Med Rehabil 62: 542
20. Fox EJ, Melzack R (1976) Transcutaneous electrical stimulation and acupuncture: comparison of treatment for low back pain. Pain 2: 141–148
21. Friedman H, Nashold BS, Somjen G (1974) Physiological effects of dorsal column stimulation. Adv Neurol 4: 769–773
22. Galetti R, Procacci PC (1966) The role of the sympathetic nervous system in the control of somatic pain and associated phenomena. Acta Neuroveg 28: 495–500
23. Goldstein A, Hilgard ERI (1975) Failure of opiate antagonist naloxone to modify hypnotic analgesia. Proc Acad Sci (Wash) 72: 2041–2043
24. Han JS, Li SJ, Tang J (1981) Tolerance to electroacupuncture and its crosstolerance to morphine. Pharmacology 20: 593–596
25. Han JS, Terenius L (1982) Neurochemical basis of acupuncture analgesia. Annu Rev Pharmacol Toxicol 22: 193–220
26. Holaday JW (1983) Cardiovascular effects of endogenous opiate systems. Annu Rev Pharmacol Toxicol 23: 541–594

27. Holmgren E (1975) Increase of pain threshold as a function of conditioning electrical stimulation. An experimental study with application to electroacupuncture for pain suppression. Am J Chin Med 3: 133–142
28. Kaada B (1985) Mechanisms of vasodilatation evoked by transcutaneous nerve stimulation (TNS). Acupunct Electrother Res 10: 217–219
29. Katz RL, Kao CY, Spiegel H, Katz GJ (1974) Pain, acupuncture, hypnosis. Adv Neurol 4: 819–825
30. Kavaliers M (1982) Pineal mediation of the thermoregulatory and behavioral activity effects of β-endorphin. Peptides 3: 679–685
31. Keppel G (1982) Design and analysis: a research handbook. Prentice-Hall, Englewood Cliffs, pp 276–332
32. Kirk RE (1968) Experimental design: procedures for the behavioral sciences. Wadsworth, Belmont, p 87
33. Kroger WS (1973) Acupunctural analgesia: its explanation by conditioning theory, autogenic training, and hypnosis. Am J Psychol 130: 855–860
34. Le Bars D, Dickenson AH, Besson JM (1979) Diffuse noxious inhibitory controls (DNIC): II. Lack of effect on non-convergent neurones, supra-spinal involvement and theoretical implications. Pain 6: 305–327
35. Lee DC, Lee MO, Clifford DH (1974) Cardiovascular effects of acupuncture in anesthetized dogs. Am J Chin Med 2: 271–282
36. Lee GT (1974) A study of electrical stimulation of acupuncture locus Tsusanli (St36) on mesenteric microcirculation. Am J Chin Med 2: 53–66
37. Lee MHM, Ernst M (1983) The sympatholytic effect of acupuncture as evidenced by thermography: a preliminary report. Orthop Rev 12: 62–72
37a. Lee MHM, Teng P, Zaretsky HH, Rubin M (1973) Acupuncture anesthesia in dentistry: a clinical investigation. NY State Dent J 39: 299–301
38. Lee MH, Sadove MS, Kim SI (1976) Liquid crystal thermography in acupuncture therapy. J Acupunct 4: 145–148
39. Lee MHM, Zaretsky HH, Ernst M, Dworkin B, Jonas R (1985) The analgesic effect of aspirin and placebo on experimentally induced tooth pulp pain. J Med 16: 417–428
40. Levine JD, Gordon NC, Fields HC (1978) The mechanisms of placebo analgesia. Lancet 2: 654–657
41. Levine JD, Gormley J, Fields HL (1976) Observations on the analgesic effects of needle puncture (acupuncture). Pain 2: 149–159
42. Lynn B, Perl ER (1977) Failure of acupuncture to produce localized analgesia. Pain 3: 339–351
43. Mayer DJ, Price DD (1976) Central nervous system mechanisms of analgesia. Pain 2: 379–404
44. Mayer DJ, Price DD, Rafii A (1977) Antagonism of acupuncture analgesia in man by the narcotic antagonist naloxone. Brain Res 121: 368–372
45. Melzack R, Wall PD (1965) Pain mechanisms: a new theory. Science 150: 971–979
46. Moore NE, Berk SN (1976) Acupuncture for chronic shoulder pain: an experimental study with attention to the role of placebo and hypnotic susceptibility. Ann Intern Med 48: 381–384
47. Nasrallah HA, Holley TY, Janowsky DS (1979) Opiate antagonism fails to reverse hypnotic induced analgesia. Lancet 1: 1355
48. Oliveras JL, Sierralta F, Fardin V, Besson JM (1981) Implication des systems serotoninergiques dans l'analgesie induite par stimulation électrique de certaines structures du tronc cérébral. J Physiol (Paris) 77: 473–482
49. Omura Y (1978) Editorial. Pain threshold measurement before and after acupuncture: controversial results of radiant heat method and electrical method. The role of ACTH-like substances and endorphins. Acupunct Electrother Res 3: 1–21
50. Omura Y (1976) Pathophysiology of acupuncture treatment: effects of acupuncture on cardiovascular and nervous systems I. Acupunct Electrother Res 1: 51–141
51. Pomeranz B, Cheng R, Law P (1977) Acupuncture reduces electrophysiological and behavioral responses to noxious stimuli: pituitary is implicated. Exp Neurol 54: 172–178
52. Procacci P, Fancini F, Maresca M, Zoppi M (1979) Skin potential and EMG changes induced by cutaneous electrical stimulation. Appl Neurophysiol 42: 125–134

53. Rosenfeld JP, Keresztes-Nagy P (1980) Differential effects of intracerebrally microinjected enkephalin analogs on centrally versus peripherally induced pain, and evidence for a facial versus lower body analgesic effect. Pain 9: 171-181
54. Sawynok J, Pinsky C, LaBella FS (1979) Mini-review on the specificity of naloxone as an opiate antagonist. Life Sci 25: 1621-1632
55. Shanghai Acupuncture Anesthesia Coordinating Group Acupuncture Anesthesia (1975) An anesthesic method combining traditional medicine and Western medicine. Chin Med J [Engl] 1: 13-27
56. Sija L, Jian T, Jisheng H (1982) The implication of central serotonin in electroacupuncture tolerance in rats. Sci Sin [B] 25: 620-629
57. Sjolund B, Eriksson M (1979) Endorphins and analgesia produced by peripheral conditioning stimulation. In: Bonica JJ, Liebeskind JC, Albe-Fessard D (eds) Advances in pain research and therapy, vol 3. Raven, New York, pp 587-592
58. Sjolund B, Terenius L, Erikson M (1977) Increased cerebrospinal fluid levels of endorphins after acupuncture. Acta Physiol Scand 100: 382-384
59. Snyder SH, Childers SR (1979) Opiate receptors and opioid peptides. Annu Rev Neurosci 2: 35-64
60. Sternbach RA (1968) Pain: a psychophysiological analysis. Academic, New York, p 185
61. Toda K, Ichioka M (1970) Electroacupuncture: relations between forelimb afferents impulses and suppression of jaw-opening reflex in the rat. Exp Neurol 61: 465-470
62. Uematsu S, Uematsu DM (1976) Thermography in chronic pain. In: Uematsu S (ed) Medical thermography. Theory and applications. Brentwood, Los Angeles, pp 52-68
63. Wall PD, Sweet WH (1967) Temporary abolition of pain in man. Science 155: 108-109
64. Wexler CE, Faanos L (1982) Lumbar, thoracic and cervical thermography. Progress in clinical biological research 1, 107: 377-388
65. Wolff BB, Horland AA (1967) Effect of suggestion upon experimental pain: a validation study. J Abn Psychol 72: 43-56
66. Wong TM, Koo A, Li CH (1981) β-endorphin. Vasodilating effect on the microcirculatory system of hamster cheek pouch. Int J Pept Protein Res 18: 420-422

Studies Supporting the Concept of Physiological Acupuncture

George A. Ulett

St. Louis University School of Medicine and Department of Psychiatry, Deaconess Hospital, 6150 Oakland Avenue, St. Louis, MO 63139, USA

Summary

The rapidly increasing amount of scientific research now permits an explanation of acupuncture mechanisms on a physiological basis. Research has shown that many useful acupuncture points are motor points, trigger points, and locations of nerves. They can be located by the use of skin potential recordings. Such knowledge has permitted the development of a simplified, anatomically based practice of acupuncture. Research has shown that electrical stimulation of these points is an effective agent for reducing experimental pain. Electroacupuncture has also been effective in relieving chronic pain in patients with a variety of medical conditions. Hypnotic suggestibility does not account for this effectiveness. Cold pressor pain is a valuable and reliable research tool for measuring the effectiveness of analgesic agents. The analgesic effect of acupuncture was unrelated to anxiety level, patient selection, prior education, suggestion or distraction, which are generally implicated in the reduction of pain utilizing methods other than drugs.

Introduction

Acupuncture has been practised in the Orient for many centuries. Its action is usually explained in terms of prescientific theories as expounded in the ancient text, *Nei Ching*. When acupuncture burst upon the scene of Western medicine in 1972, American physicians were skeptical of the meridian theory. They felt that acupuncture had no physical basis. The American Medical Association officially refused to accept acupuncture, and doctors who witnessed surgery with acupuncture as the analgesic agent labelled it as "Oriental hypnosis." The National Institutes of Health set up a committee to investigate acupuncture, and my group of investigators received the first grant given for such purposes. Initially, we sought to determine whether acupuncture points had a real existence. Later, these points were used to control both experimental and clinical pain. The effect of acupuncture and hypnosis as modifiers for pain control was studied.

Traditionally, acupuncture needles have been stimulated by twirling. In order to increase their effectiveness, moxibustion was added. The use of electricity for stimulation of acupuncture needles was first reported in Japan. Its application has spread widely so that at present it is a standard method for stimulation. Needling with and without electrical stimulation was compared and electroacupuncture, hypnosis, and morphine sulfate were found to reduce pain between 40% and 50%. Needling without electrical stimulation was much less effective.

These studies began in the laboratory with an investigation of how to locate acupuncture points accurately. We then looked at the results of acupuncture stimulation, first upon the white cell count and body temperature and then its effectiveness in the control of experimental pain. This method of pain control was compared with that achieved by hypnosis. We then moved to the more difficult task of comparing acupuncture pain control and the control of pain by hypnosis in patients who had experienced acupuncture treatments for clinical conditions with chronic pain. The results of such studies were encouraging, so the techniques were brought into clinical practice. We have now had over 10 years of experience in the treatment of chronic pain by electroacupuncture. Recently some treatments have combined electroacupuncture with hypnosis.

The text, *Principles and Practice of Physiologic Acupuncture,* presents this method of simplified, anatomically based technique of acupuncture. It has been useful in the teaching of medical students.

Location of Points

Traditionally, acupuncture points are located along hypothetical meridian channels as depicted on ancient charts [1]. They are described in relationship to external anatomical landmarks from which they are measured in terms of "cun". The cun or "Chinese inch" is described as the distance between the skin creases seen in the partially bent middle finger from the proximal end of the first phalanx and the distal end of the third phalanx. This, of course, varies with the size of each person's body, size of the hands, etc. Due to variations in bone length, muscle mass, etc., the several hundred points shown on acupuncture charts give, at best, only approximate locations. It is said that trained acupuncturists identify location through palpation techniques and the patient's objective responses to needling. To avoid such subjective variances emphasis was laid on a study of points with differing electrical characteristics located at random on the skin [2]. Devices (point finders) which measure changes in skin resistance are now commonly sold as a means for the location of acupuncture points. This method requires the application of electricity to the skin to measure its resistance to the passage of the current. The results of these brief efforts using the resistance technique suggest that with repeated application of a probe to a single skin site, the amplitude of the response (in millivolts) decreases with each trial until the site no longer gives a physical response. The implication is that the electrical resistance of the skin site had become elevated to the passage of the small currents. The currents were no longer effective in penetrating the skin at this site, thus there was no drop in skin resistance observed as compared to surrounding nonacupuncture points.

For these reasons the skin was explored using potential recording techniques for the identification and mapping of acupuncture loci. Such skin potentials depend solely on the electricity generated by the body itself. The outer skin surface is electrically negative with respect to the subcutaneous tissue, and the potential differences are measured in millivolts (mV).

(LEFT ARM, REAR VIEW)

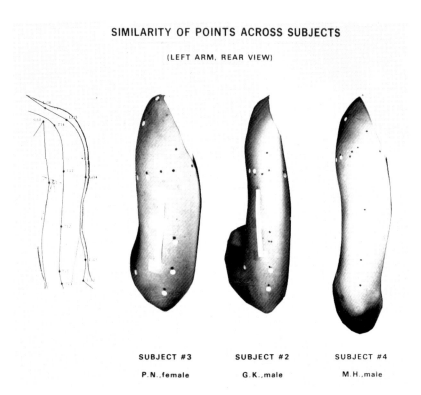

SUBJECT #3   SUBJECT #2   SUBJECT #4

P.N.,female   G.K.,male   M.H.,male

Fig. 1. The *black circles* on the subjects' arms indicate the points located by this method. As a guide, we used charts of traditional loci shown in the drawings at the *extreme left of top and bottom rows* [1]. These drawings show the meridianal pathways on which the loci are said to be located. The *outer line (LI)* is the large intestine meridian; the *center line (TB)* is called triple burner meridian; the *inner line* is the small intestine *(SI)* meridian

The upper arms of eight healthy volunteers were searched blindly for points from which large potential differences were elicited (Fig. 1). These points were then compared with the acupuncture points shown on the traditional charts.

The device employed to locate the points on the skin consisted of a hand-held probe connected to a high input-impedence direct current amplifier. The probe was a solid (jewelers) silver bar, 10 cm long, 3 mm wide, and 1 mm thick, with its probe tip rounded to 2 mm in diameter while the opposite end of the bar was connected to the one megohme DC input of the polygraph with both the metal shield of the cable and the indifferent electrode connected to ground. The reference (inactive), electrode was placed on the contralateral arm to the one being searched. A reference area was located on the volar surface of the upper forearm about 5 cm below the elbow crease along its inner edge. The site was cleaned with alcohol and "skin drilled" according to the method of Shackel [3]. An Ag-AgCl electrode filled with electrode jelly was applied to the site with an adhesive collar.

The pen recorder was calibrated to give a pen deflection of 1 mV/cm; an upward pen deflection indicated a potential of increasing negativity. When the probe was lightly held on acupuncture loci, the pen deflected from the center line,

179

ADJACENT POINTS ON MERIDIAN
SHOWING DIFFERENT POLARITY AND DIFFERENT AMPLITUDE

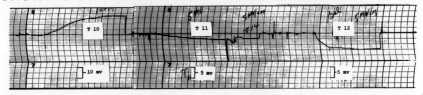

Fig. 2. Different polarity and amplitude of DC voltage shown by adjacent 3 points on a meridian with respect to control skin. *Down* is positive, *up* is negative, *T10* was −17 mV; *T11* was +3 mV; and *T12* was −8 mV

and when the asymptote (maximum amplitude) was approached the pen would remain at this amplitude until the probe was removed from the skin. Most of the potential recording reported in this study was obtained with a "dry active electrode," i.e., no electrode paste used between the skin and the roving electrode.

By this method eighteen discreet loci were located on the upper arm. These included all loci on the upper arm shown on the acupuncture charts as well as a few loci not listed on such charts. All of these loci produce responses of potential differences ranging from 2–42 mV. Symmetry of point location was observed between the right and left arms of the same subject. Differences between the two arms and the location of similar loci from common references range between 0 and 3.5 cm for all subjects. Wide variations in amplitude potential response for adjacent loci along single meridians were found (Fig. 2). A decrease in skin potential implied that the "active" site was less "negative" with respect to the reference electrode in the surrounding tissue. Increasing negativity produced an upward deflection, and decreasing negativity produced a downward deflection. A third type of response was bipolar in form (Fig. 3). The most common response observed was a decrease in negative potential (downward deflection). Some 80% of the responses from the left arm and 89% of the responses from the right arm were of this nature. Another 6% and 3%, respectively, demonstrated increases in negative potential, and the remaining trials showed mixed responses. The loci remained stable over a period of time with respect to location, and, equally important, there was little or no change in amplitude of potential response at each site during the 3-h time lapse.

This study thus suggests that, at least for the upper arm, one can identify stable, electrically active loci, which are bilaterally symmetrical and include those points identified and utilized by acupuncturists. The skin potential procedure is a reliable technique for the precise location of acupuncture loci.

Although this method of location was used initially in our research work, we slowly came to the realization that useful acupuncture loci were simply points at which one could obtain access to the peripheral nervous system. The work of Liu [4] clearly suggests that many useful points are often the motor points used by electromyographers as the best place to elicit nerve stimulation (Fig. 4). Gun [5] added Golgi tendon organs to this concept. In clinical work needles were also often placed close to the point of nerve exit, as in the case of treating problems

180

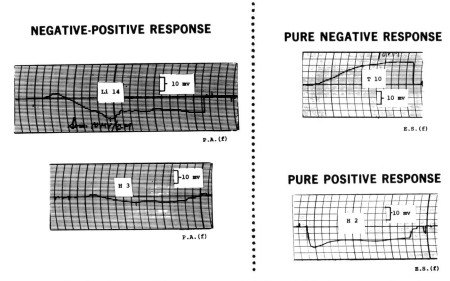

NEGATIVE-POSITIVE RESPONSE

Li 14   10 mv

P.A.(f)

H 3   10 mv

P.A.(f)

PURE NEGATIVE RESPONSE

T 10   10 mv

E.S.(f)

PURE POSITIVE RESPONSE

H 2   10 mv

E.S.(f)

Fig. 3. Types of resting skin potential at acupuncture loci *Upward deflections* are negative voltages and *downward* are positive

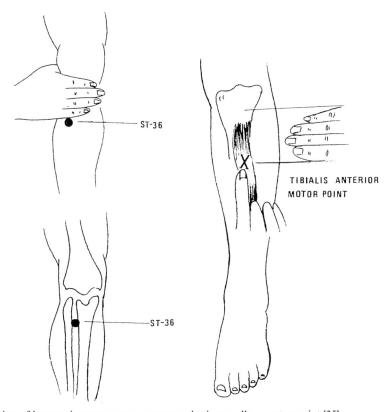

ST-36

ST-36

TIBIALIS ANTERIOR
MOTOR POINT

Fig. 4. Illustration of how an important acupuncture point is actually a motor point [35]

181

with the trigeminal nerve. Using the principle of neurotomes, points were selected adjacent to the exit of spinal nerves on the posterior surface of the trunk. With electrical stimulation of needles, such a rule of thumb is sufficient for locating points for needle insertion because simply raising the amplitude of the electrical stimulus can overcome any slight inaccuracy of needle placement.

Effect of Acupuncture on the White Cell Count

We next turned out attention to the effect of needling on the white blood cell count in normal healthy male volunteers [6]. Cheng [7] has shown that needling certain points of the body of a normal person or animal increased phagocytosis. This statement is also found in a book by P. Chan [8] and in studies conducted at the General Hospital of Kwang Chow, China [9]. Cracium et al. studied white cell counts before and after needling of the acupuncture point Du 14 Dazhui, below the 7th cervical vertebra, in groups of normal, healthy, volunteer students and reported increases in white cell counts of 59% in one study [10] and 44% in the other [11].

Twelve healthy, normal, male volunteers ranging in age from 19 to 29 years were used. The white blood cell count can increase up to 60% within 12 h of eating foods to which one has been found to be "allergic" by the Cytotoxic Food Test [12]. Thus, all subjects had to refrain from eating, drinking, or smoking for a minimum of 6 h prior to testing. The white blood cell count was examined the day before, during, and after the electrical stimulation of four well-known acupuncture sites as well as in four areas that showed no electrical evidence of containing acupuncture points. The method of locating the acupuncture sites on the skin surface was through the use of skin potential measurements as previously described. The stimuli used for all subjects were 20 min of sawtooth pulses of 100 Hz frequency, a duration of pulses of 0.02 ms, and voltages ranging from 1 to 30 V. Following the insertion of acupuncture needles the first blood sample was drawn from a fingertip on the subject's right hand. This blood was for the pre-stimulation baseline. After this the stimulation was begun on the needles of the left arm. The subject's task was to tell the experimenter the moment he felt any sensation at the site being stimulated. The intensity would then be slowly increased until a strong but not painful sensation was felt at the needle site. When all four needles were felt to be strongly but not painfully stimulated, the time was recorded for the start of a 20-min period of stimulation. After 5 min of stimulation the second blood sample was taken from the right hand, with a third sample taken immediately upon termination of the stimulation. At this time the stimulator was turned off, and the leads and the needles were removed. Fifteen minutes after the cessation of stimulation a fourth blood sample was taken, with a fifth and final sample taken 10 min later. Skin temperature was recorded at 5-min intervals throughout each investigation.

After needle insertion and while probing for the location of the acupuncture points, there was a slight increase in the white blood cell count. This suggested that Pavlov's "expectancy response" was operative here. Needle insertion had a negligible effect on blood cell count even with needles remaining in place for as long as 90–120 min (Fig. 5). The greatest response, however, was seen with electri-

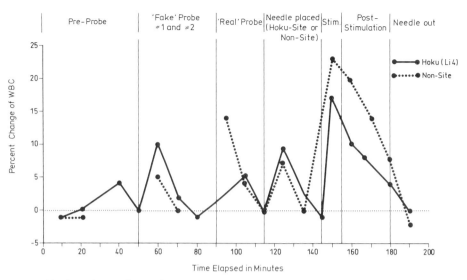

Fig. 5. Absolute changes in WBC count associated with specific events. WBC count was allowed to return to baseline before introducing the succeeding event. For one subject, the baseline for Hegu needling is 8150 cells/mm³; for another subject, single, "non-site" needling leads to 6650 cells/mm³

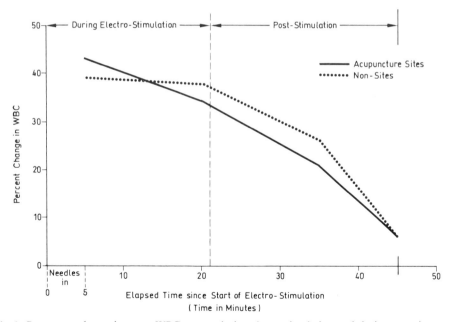

Fig. 6. Percentage change in mean WBC counts during electrostimulation and during poststimulation with needles removed. Post-needling mean WBC baseline was 7408 cells/mm³ for nine subjects with acupuncture site placements and 8036 cells/mm³ for seven subjects with "non-site" placements

183

cal stimulation whether it was or was not at an acupuncture site. This procedure evoked the largest increase in white blood cell count of all procedures measured. Regardless of the nature of the event, a decrease in white blood cell count then occurred over time. Even 35-45 min after stimulation the white blood cell count was still declining to the base level (Fig.6).

The most significant finding from the verbal reports comparing site versus non-site data was that 69% of the subjects reported feeling pain from the needles, both on insertion and while the needle remained embedded in the tissue of non-site placements. Only 17% of subjects reported feeling pain from needles placed in acupuncture sites. Pain did not relate to the electrical stimulation.

As shown by these data, the effects of emotional or psychological factors in increasing white blood cell count are equally as important as needle insertion, and their effectiveness is exceeded only after 5-20 min of electrical stimulation of the needle. If such factors are not taken into account and their effect not cancelled by allowing time for the cell count to return to the baseline, an incorrect count is obtained by accumulating subsequent increases. This effect of psychological factors has been reported by others [13].

The white blood cell response as seen from these studies appears to be a nonspecific response as a result of the procedure of needling in acupuncture or non-acupuncture sites.

Acupuncture, Hypnosis in Experimental Pain (Normal volunteers)

It has been suggested that acupuncture effects are mediated principally through suggestibility and/or hypnosis [14, 15]. Most of the anesthetic and analgesic effects claimed for acupuncture stimulation, both manual and electrical, can also be brought about with hypnosis [16]. This portion of the study was designed to explore the analgesic effects of electroacupuncture as compared with hypnosis and a number of pharmacological agents. The experiments were designed to answer the question of whether the analgesic effect of electroacupuncture on experimentally induced pain could be attributable entirely to suggestibility or hypnotizability.

This study employed 20 normal, healthy, Caucasian males, aged 18-30 years, who volunteered as paid subjects. Pain was produced by one of two methods. In the first, a cold bath was maintained by refrigeration at 0 °C. A plastic sheet was placed across the surface of the water, thus permitting the subject's left forearm to remain dry while only the fingers were immersed the cold water. The intensity of the cold experience was, thus, considerably less than that found in standard cold pressor tests where the arm was fully immersed. The second type of pain, pressure pain, was produced by means of a sphygmomanometer attached to a blood pressure cuff placed around the subject's left arm at the level of the biceps with the cuff inflated to 300 mm Hg and held steady at that level by a clamp. The challenging agents employed to alter the experimentally induced pain were (a) hypnosis, (b) electrostimulation of acupuncture points, (c) electrostimulation of nonpoints, and (d) the drugs morphine, aspirin, diazepam, and placebo. In each session the subject was exposed twice to the painful stimulus, once under control without any modifying agents such as drugs or acupuncture (herewith called "control pain") and once under the experimental conditions. The order of the challenging agents and the two pain induction procedures (cuff or cold) was randomized. Six physiological variables, EEG, EKG, EMG, skin temperature, peripheral vascular activity, and respiration, were sampled under the various conditions. Hypnosis induction was achieved by means of a standardized video tape recording viewed by the subject on a TV monitor. Stimulation was from a Grass model S-4 stimulator through the acupuncture needles. A common indifferent electrode (EKG plate) was placed with a rubber strap on the subject's left inner wrist. The electrical stimulation was at a frequency of 130 Hz. Current output was 10 mA maximum (pulse amplitude), and pulse wave forms were square. Pulse duration was 0.1 ms and biphasic in form. Duration of the stimulation through the needles was standardized to 50 min. Acupuncture true loci and random false loci were determined using the skin potential method previously described.

At each 15-s interval during the 5-min pain period for both cold and pressure pain, subjects were asked to signal intensity of the pain via a finger switch connected to the channel of the polygraph, their rating of the degree of pain experienced, and these were recorded using a 5-point scale: zero meaning no pain, 1 mild pain, 2 moderate pain, and 3 severe pain. Stimulus was stopped at the subjects' request when it was no longer tolerable, and a score of 4 was entered for each 15-s interval of the time remaining in the 5-min pain period.

All hypnosis subjects were screened using Form A of the Harvard Group Scale for Hypnotic Suggestibility prior to their first experimental session. Volunteers were administered this scale until a group of 20 subjects who completed all 14 of the experiments was gathered. Drug dosages used were: morphine sulfate, intramuscularly in the right arm, 10 mg/70 kg of body weight; diazepam, 10 mg in a 2-ml solution intravenously; aspirin, two tablets of 75 mg each given orally; and two small white capsules resembling Darvon (propoxyphene) but containing milk sugar were given orally as the placebo. Fig. 7 summarizes the results obtained.

It was found from higher mean scores on both trials that the cold baths were a more painful experience than the inflating of the cuff. The difference between control and experimental pain scores was tested by t-tests. It was found that acupuncture with electrical stimulation at true loci was an effective pain reliever for cold bath pain ($P < 0.01$). This failed to reach the 0.05 level of significance on cuff trials ($P < 0.065$). Hypnosis provided the most effective analgesia for both types of pain, cold bath ($P < 0.001$) and cuff ($P < 0.001$). Morphine produced an analgesic effect similar to acupuncture on both types of pain, cold bath ($P < 0.02$) and cuff ($P < 0.001$). None of the other four challenges, acupuncture at false loci, diazepam, aspirin, or placebo, showed effectiveness as pain relievers.

Results on some of the physiological variables were as follows: For analgesia by both hypnosis and acupuncture at true sites, electrical stimulation produced the highest resting heart rates. The EMG showed a greater basal activity after both true and false electrical stimulation under the cold pressor conditions during control pain.

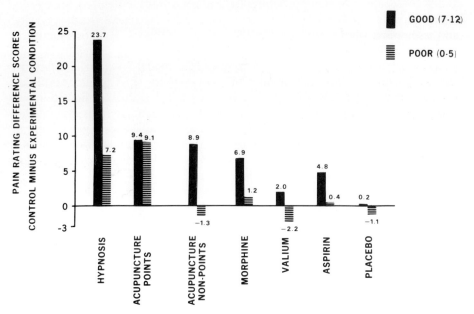

PAIN RATING (DIFFERENCE) COLD PRESSOR

COMPARISON OF 'GOOD' & 'POOR' HYPNOTIC SUBJECTS (HARVARD SCALE)

Fig. 7. Cold pressor results: 20 subjects were given 7 types of analgesic treatments in random order and were tested for cold pressor and cuff ischemic pain. This graph shows cold pressor results

Conclusion

It was found that acupuncture with electrical stimulation of true sites specifically reduced experimental pain induced by a cold bath when compared with controlled trials without acupuncture. Electroacupuncture of true sites also caused some analgesia with cuff pain, but this did not reach significance, perhaps due to the low intensity of this type of pain (cold bath produced more severe pain than the cuff). Thus, it appears from both these data and those of other experiments that acupuncture is an effective challenger of experimentally induced pain.

No significant pain relief was derived from false site (sham) electrical stimulation as compared with controls for either cold pressor or ischemic pain. It has been suggested by some that analgesia could be a function of reduced anxiety. During these experiments it was noticed that the integrated EMG showed higher basal activity both during true and false site electrical stimulation during the cold pressor trials, suggesting that the analgesia produced by acupuncture is unrelated to the anxiety level of the subject. The increased heart beat after true site stimulation also strengthens this argument.

186

Acupuncture, Hypnosis in Chronic Pain Patients
(Reaction to Experimental Pain)

Study Description

Twenty patients with a history of chronic pain were subjected to cold water-induced pain (cold pressor pain), and the data on the effect of 35 min of hypnotic suggestion and 20 min of acupuncture stimulation on the pain and other physiological variables were gathered in a controlled setting. These patients had previously had acupuncture treatment. Eleven had benefitted from acupuncture treatments in excess of 50% while nine had reported less than 50% improvement in their condition. This experiment was designed to determine retrospectively the predictability of outcome with acupuncture treatment. The subjects selected had been in active treatment by means of acupuncture for basically similar conditions using traditionally selected acupuncture points.

Patients with chronic low back pain and knee pain were chosen. These patients were selected from this clinic where a number of patients with these conditions have been treated over a 3-year period. From case records, all patients with back and knee pain were selected regardless of treatment outcome, of which 45 cases fitted these criteria. The first 20 patients accepting were recruited into the study. Patients were not paid, but all were offered an additional course of acupuncture treatment without cost. Patients ranged in age from 2 to 70 years. There were 9 females and 11 males with an average duration of pain of 8 years. All had been treated unsuccessfully by other physicians with tranquillizers and analgesics. After an initial examination, informed consent was obtained, and subjects were advised that they would undergo an experimental study in two sessions, one with hypnosis and one with acupuncture. The settings were to be determined on a random basis. Four acupuncture points on the arm which were used in previous experimental studies were selected. These were LI.4, LI.11, LI.14, and LI.15, all of which had been reliably noted to have produced analgesia in the hand. These points corresponded to commonly identified trigger points. They were stimulated by means of a Grass Model 4 stimulator. Stimulator intensity for each needle was monitored by a Tektronix differential oscilloscope. Stimulation was given at 130 Hz, 10 mA maximum (pulse amplitude), and with a pulse duration of 1 ms. Acupuncture points were located by the method of skin potential as previously described. With each 15-s interval during the 5-min period the subject was asked to signal the degree of pain by moving a finger switch which produced a recording on one channel of the polygraph. Pain was rated using a 5-point scale with 0 indicating no pain, 1 mild pain, 2 moderate pain, and 3 severe pain. If the pain became intolerable the pain stimulator was stopped at the request of the subject, the hand was removed from the bath, and the rating was recorded as 4.

The experiment proceeded as follows: (a) rest periods of 10 min after location of acupuncture sites, (b) control pain induction and rating for 5 min, (c) needle insertion with stimulation for 20 min, (d) experimental pain induction and rating for 5 min, and (e) rest for 10 min.

The effects of suggestibility and its possible predictive value in terms of the usefulness of hypnosis in preventing noxious perception were of interest in this investigation. A short version of instructions for the Harvard Group Scale [17] was used to evaluate hypnotic suggestibility. The instructions were recorded on magnetic tape, and subjects listened to the tape prior to filling out the scale. The scheme for the hypnosis experiment was as follows: (a) 10-min rest period, (b) 5-min controlled pain rating, and (c) 35 min of videotaped induction and hypnosis using task motivation and instructions by Barber and Halverly [18] (a videotaped hypnosis induction procedure was used to ensure uniformity; this procedure is well tested and appears to be as good as direct therapists' instruction [4, 19]), (d) 5-min experimental pain rating, (e) 20 min deepening of trace and evaluation of trace using Barber Suggestibility Scale (both d and e were done with video instructions), and (f) 10 min of rest. The patients who participated in this study had been treated with acupuncture therapy and as part of their progress notes had been asked at the end of each treatment period to evaluate the degree of improvement in their condition over the treatment period. Seventeen of the 20 patients were seen by different acupuncture therapists. If a patient or the therapist at either period rated the patient as improved by 50%, 75%, or 100%, then they were classified as acupuncture therapy responsive. If improvement was rated 25% or 0% they were classified as nonresponsive. On this basis, 11 patients were responsive and 9 were nonresponsive.

The various data were then analyzed according to the four different conditions of research: (1) suggestible and nonsuggestible populations, (2) acupuncture responsive and nonresponsive populations, (3) suggestible acupuncture responsive and suggestible acupuncture nonresponsive populations, and (4) nonsuggestible acupuncture responsive and nonsuggestible acupuncture nonresponsive populations.

All patients were exposed to the pain four times on two occasions, including a control period required of each hypnosis and acupuncture experiment. The data were analyzed using analysis of variance techniques with four dependent variables: (1) groups (acupuncture responsive and nonresponsive patients), (2) treatment (hypnosis and acupuncture), (3) manipulation (cold pressor technique under control and cold pressor technique during the two treatment conditions), and (4) the interaction between treatment and manipulation of the patient (i.e., during cold pressor application).

Results

The results demonstrate a significant group effect, with acupuncture responsive patients demonstrating less pain under all conditions and a significant treatment by manipulation effect. It also appeared that there were differences in age between the two groups. The average age of responsive patients was 54.09 years, while that for the poor responders was 66.89 years. Differences between these groups were significant.

The correlation between performance on the Harvard Group Hypnotizability Scale and the pain reduction by hypnosis was high indicating that those who had the highest scores on measured hypnotic suggestibility obtained the greatest relief from pain when exposed to it under hypnosis.

188

The data suggest that acupuncture and hypnosis are distinct and independent treatment modes; that since hypnotic susceptibility does not predict success with acupuncture treatment. Our results show that acupuncture responsive patients have higher thresholds of pain and perceive it less than the average population and that acupuncture may be useful in younger populations.

Electrophysiological Changes

Sensory Evoked Potential

Twenty mentally and physically healthy male volunteers with an age range of 19–34 years (mean 35 years) and a weight range of 58–89 kg (mean 72 kg) participated in the study [20]. Pain was induced by somatic sensory stimuli designed for eliciting somatosensory evoked potentials (SEP), consisting of brief electrical stimuli applied at 2-s intervals over the median nerve with a pulse duration of 0.1 ms. Actually, the stimuli were not really painful since their intensity ranged from 35–80 V depending upon the subject's threshold (threshold plus 50%). Stimuli were produced by an especially designed constant voltage stimulator triggered by a Tektronix 162 wave form generator and Tektronix 161 pulse generator. Their output was fed into a Grass stimulus isolation unit (model SIU-4B) connected to the subject's right wrist by means of two, 8-mm diameter, silver electrodes which were 3 cm apart (anode distal). A ground electrode was placed proximal to the cathode. Twice in each session (before and during analgesia) 250 stimuli were applied (each session lasting approximately 9 min).

The pain challengers included hypnosis, acupuncture, and analgesic drugs. In two sessions, "hypno-analgesia" was induced by videotape [19]. The principal difference was the identity of the hypnotist. There were four acupuncture sessions. In the first the needles were inserted at specific loci as recommended by Chinese medicine for analgesia of the wrist, LI.4 and LI.7, and in the second session needles were placed at nonspecific sites near the specific loci. In the third session the subject filled out a self-rating scale.

Neurophysiological parameters included: quantitatively analyzed 5-min resting EEG recordings (RR) and 9-min SEP and concomitant EEG (SEP/EEG) recordings. The specific recording SEP leads were placed in a parasagittal plane 7 cm to the left and right of the midline. The posterior electrode was placed 2 cm behind the line from the vertex to the external auditory meatus and the anterior was placed 7 cm in front of the posterior electrode. In addition, a reading from the right and left occipital leads with reference electrodes at the ears was recorded. A ground electrode was placed on the forehead. SEPs and EEGs were recorded and amplified by a Grass polygraph model 79 and Ampex FR 1300 tape recorder. SEPs were fed into a CAT 400 B for summation. Analysis time was 500 ms. Each average SEP to 250 stimuli was plotted on a Moseley XY plotter. The EEG was analyzed off-line utilizing EEG digital computer analysis programs [21, 22]. This method permits analysis of 22 EEG parameters (including average frequency, frequency deviation, and eight different frequency bands of each of the primary and first derivative waves), as well as the average absolute amplitude and the amplitude variability (Drohocki measurements) at a sampling rate of 320 points per second. Any 10-s epoch demonstrating movement or muscle artifacts was excluded from statistical analysis.

The temporal ordering was constant for each session starting with a 5-min resting record and a 9-min SEP/EEG recording. Then the pain challenger was applied. Nineteen minutes after the start of hypnosis, acupuncture, or saline injection, a 5-min "analgesia" resting record was obtained. An 8-min pause followed, and subsequently, the "analgesia" SEP/EEG was recorded for 9 min (32 min after application of the pain challenger). In the morphine session the "analgesia" resting record was not started until 27 min after injection because the drug effect peaks 1 h after IM administration while the SEP/EEG record was started as usual, at 32 min after the injection. In the ketamine trials the time sequence was changed because of the rapid onset of drug action. The "analgesia" resting record was started at 4 min after the injection, and the SEP/EEG recording followed immediately thereafter.

Statistical analysis of the stimulus intensity ratings demonstrated a significant decrease in the subjective experience of pain after the application of several pain challengers. In each subject the SEP stimulus intensity was kept the same during both the prerecordings as well as the analgesia recordings.

With insertion of acupuncture needles in specific loci, only a slight and insignificant decrease was noted (from 1.7 to 1.5). However, electroacupuncture of the same specific sites resulted in a significant ($P<0.01$) decrease of pain (from 1.7 to 1.3). When the needles were inserted at nonacupuncture points, no change in the pain experience occurred. Electroacupuncture in unspecific loci did not result in any particular change (from 1.5 to 1.4). Morphine sulfate administered IM produced a significant ($P<0.01$) decrease in the perceived stimulus intensity. Ketamine was administered at two different doses due to the fact that despite an intensive literature search no data could be obtained indicating which dosage would be analgesic in adults and which would be anesthetic. Thus, nine subjects received 5 mg per kg. It turned out that this dosage was anesthetic as the subjects did not respond to external stimuli. Anesthesia was reached approximately 6 min after injection and lasted for 20 min.

The decrease in the perceived stimulus intensity with hypnosis I and hypnosis II was significant ($P<0.01$) as compared with the control session, during which the pain experience did not change. Over four acupuncture sessions only electroacupuncture at specific (real) loci elicited a significant response ($P<0.01$) or attenuation of feeling the stimulus intensity. This attenuation was only slightly below that experienced with hypnosis and morphine. Morphine was significantly different from the control session ($P<0.05$). Hypnosis I and hypnosis II were significantly more effective in reducing pain than acupuncture at specific loci with and without electrical stimulation. Morphine was only significantly superior to acupuncture at unspecific loci in the control session. No comparison between ketamine and other conditions was made due to its anesthetic effect which precluded any of the subjects giving a response during the period of stimulation.

Examination of the SEP findings revealed 12 peaks identified within the first 500 ms following the stimulus. Peaks 1 and 2 can be regarded as the primary evoked response ("sensory response"), while the subsequent peaks can be looked upon as secondary response ("cognitive response"). The primary response is seen in the contralateral hemisphere (left side). Over the ipsilateral hemisphere (right side), the first two peaks were absent. The latency of each peak from the stimulus artifact and the peak-to-peak amplitudes were measured for statistical analysis.

During the control session no statistically significant alterations occurred with the exception of the amplitude increase in peaks 9–10. In contrast, during hypnotic analgesia there occurred a latency increase in the early second response that was significant ($P < 0.05$) in peak 4 on the left side and a significant latency decrease in the late response in the peak on the right side. The amplitude of the late components was attenuated and reached the level of statistical significance in peaks 7 and 8 (left side) and peaks 10 and 11 on both sides.

Acupuncture in specific loci resulted in a latency decrease in the early secondary response (significant in right-sided peaks 5 and 6), and a latency decrease in the late response (significant in right-sided peaks 8–11). In terms of amplitude, a significant decrease was observed in peaks 7 and 8 of the left side, while on the right side a significant augmentation of peaks 4 and 5 occurred. Electroacupuncture in specific loci produced a significant latency decrease in left-sided peaks 3 and 8 as well as an amplitude augmentation of peaks 3 and 4. Insertion of the needles in nonspecific loci resulted similarly in a latency increase in the early portion and a latency decrease in the late portion of the response which, however, only reached the level of statistical significance in the left-sided peak 3. There were no significant changes with electroacupuncture in nonspecific loci.

EEG Results

Computer analyzed EEG from period analysis of the resting record during the control session demonstrated no significant changes as compared with the pre-resting record. During both hypnosis sessions a significant increase of delta and theta activity as well as a significant decrease of alpha and slow beta waves (average frequency and frequency deviations) were observed. Acupuncture, with needle insertion alone at specific sites, produced only one significant effect, i.e., an increase in very high frequency activity (90 cps and above). Electroacupuncture at the same specific loci resulted in a significant attenuation of delta and beta waves ($P < 0.05$).

Acupuncture at nonspecific loci did not induce any significant alterations, while electroacupuncture at nonspecific sites produced a decrease of slow activity (significant in the delta band), an increase in the 13–20 cps beta band, and an increase in average frequency.

Acupuncture was an effective pain challenger when needles were inserted at specific loci and electrically stimulated. Insertion of the needles alone at nonspecific sites or acupuncture in specific loci without electrical stimulation did not affect pain perception nor did it affect the quantitatively analyzed EEG. Significant changes in the quantitatively analyzed EEG occurred only with electroacupuncture at specific points and were characterized by a decrease in delta and beta waves, 16–26 CPS activity, and amplitude variability as well as by an increase in average frequency for absolute amplitude alpha, slow beta waves, and very fast beta activity. Our findings are in agreement with those of the Peking Acupuncture and Anesthesia Coordinating Group [23], who found that during needling the alpha wave predominated and its amplitude increased. In our study acupuncture-induced changes were significantly different and generally opposite from the hypnosis-induced alterations. These indicated a stimulatory effect of electroacupuncture regardless of the site of stimulation.

Conclusions: Electrophysiological Changes

Interestingly, SEP changes are almost exclusively statistically significant when acupuncture needles are inserted in specific loci with and without current stimulation. After these changes a latency decrease in the early peaks 2 and 3 and very late peaks 8 and 12 and an increase in the middle portion of SEP in peaks 5 and 6 occurred. Thus, we were able to support the findings of the Peking Acupuncture Anesthesia Coordinating Group [23] who showed that needling the points LI.4 Hegu and Pe.6 Neiguan suppressed or weakened the potential evoked by painful stimulation of the nervi cutaneus colli in animals.

Neurophysiological findings, both EEG and SEP, demonstrated that electrical stimulation of acupuncture at specific loci does have a significant influence on brain activity. This is in agreement with the view of Chang Hsiang-Tung [24]. It is thus suggested that the efficacy of acupuncture analgesia may be affected by the state of brain excitability and is due to the inhibited interaction between afferent impulses arriving from the needle points and those from the sites of pain impulses in the brain, especially in the thalamus.

During both of the hypnosis sessions a significant increase in slow EEG activity occurred together with some decrease in the alpha band. In some cases there was also an increase in delta together with a decrease in beta activity. Acupuncture with needle insertion of specific sites produced a significant increase in high frequency beta activity [20].

Acupuncture Versus Hypnosis

Pronouncements were made on by two leading hypotherapists, Speigel [14] and Kroger [15], that acupuncture was a kind of Oriental hypnosis induction therapy. This opinion derived from a vast experience with hypnosis but little with acupuncture and had the "halo" effect of strengthening the widespread belief that acupuncture was merely a form of hypnosis. Increasing familiarity with acupuncture, however, led to a change of opinion. Patrick Wall, for example, stated that, "in 1972, my own belief is that acupuncture is an effective use of hypnosis" [25]. In 1974, after a tour of China, he retracted that statement [26].

Ronald Katz, who reported that a positive response to acupuncture was closely related to a high score on hypnosis susceptibility testing [27] later stated, "I have assisted in four operations under acupuncture anesthesia and many more than that under hypnosis. The patients behave differently. Those under hypnosis are in a tight self-controlled world, seemingly unaware of what is going on about them.

192

Patients under acupuncture were part of the team, joking, laughing and commenting freely" [28].

From an extensive review of the literature, Lu and Needham [29] stated that one cannot deny the importance of a certain measure of suggestion and suggestibility such as occurs in all treatments but that it is a gross misuse of the term hypnosis to cover all aspects of acupuncture treatment.

Omura [30] mentions his study of 300 patients using the Speigel Eye-Roll Hypnotizability Test. He found that those persons with hypnotizability scores above three had a slightly better response to acupuncture. Yet more than 50% of his subjects with hypnotizability scores of 0 showed beneficial effects of acupuncture treatment.

Matsumoto [31], using acupuncture both clinically and experimentally, concludes "... our clinical experience mitigates against the concept that acupuncture is a form of hypnosis." Our own experiences have been similar [32]. We did, however, observe that clinical and experimental pain are different phenomena and respond differently to acupuncture. Cold pressor pain, such as we and others have utilized in the experimental laboratory, certainly has different characteristics from the chronic pain syndromes that make up the bulk of clinical acupuncture practice. Today there is sufficient neuroanatomical and neurochemical knowledge of pain mechanisms to suggest the basis for such differences and thus to, account for some of the differing results reported.

Goldstein and Hilgard [33] in 1975 pointed out that while naloxone inhibits the analgesia of morphine and acupuncture, it does not inhibit hypnoanalgesia. Related to this in the important finding of Levine et al. [34] that naloxone blocks the placebo analgesic response that curbs the pain of electrical stimulation of tooth pulp. Thus, one must apparently differentiate between the term suggestibility as applied to placebo responders and suggestibility implying hypnotizability.

The psychological response does not predict acupuncture response. It has become increasingly clear from these investigations that hypnosis and acupuncture act in different ways upon the complex pain mechanisms within the central nervous system. Accordingly, in our clinical work with patients for whom acupuncture has failed, we have sometimes turned to hypnosis with good results. These two methods then seem complementary to each other.

In order to avoid the use of analgesic drugs with their propensity for unwanted side effects and potential for addiction, the optimal nondrug approach for the modulation of pain might well include three techniques, each with a different action component within the central nervous system: maximization of the placebo response (psychological/physiological) which is abolished by naloxone; electroacupuncture (physiological), also abolished by naloxone; and hypnosis (psychological/physiological), not abolished by naloxone.

In our study of 20 healthy volunteers using cold pressor (water bath pain), ischemic (tourniquet cuff pain) and electrical stimulation pain to elicit the SEP response, we found the protective effects of both 35 min of hypnotic suggestion and electroacupuncture stimulation at specific points to be effective methods of pain relief and at least as potent as the administration of 10 mg of morphine sulfate. Our studies found that hypnosis, electroacupuncture, and morphine sulfate were all nearly equally effective in reducing experimental pain (Fig. 8). While our

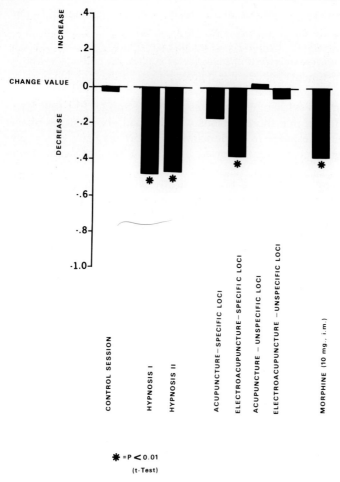

INCREASE

CHANGE VALUE

DECREASE

.4
.2
0
-.2
-.4
-.6
-.8
-1.0

✳ ✳ ✳ ✳

CONTROL SESSION

HYPNOSIS I

HYPNOSIS II

ACUPUNCTURE—SPECIFIC LOCI

ELECTROACUPUNCTURE—SPECIFIC LOCI

ACUPUNCTURE – UNSPECIFIC LOCI

ELECTROACUPUNCTURE – UNSPECIFIC LOCI

MORPHINE (10 mg., i.m.)

✳ = P < 0.01
(t-Test)

Fig. 8. Changes in the subjects' experience of experimental pain with different pain challengers (analgesics) ($n = 20$)

good hypnotic subjects did respond better to both hypnosis and electroacupuncture, we found that the poor hypnotic subjects also responded well to electroacupuncture. It was our conclusion, therefore, that electroacupuncture given at specific acupuncture points was an effective agent for reducing experimental pain and that hypnotic susceptibility does not account for this effectiveness.

In a study of 20 patients who had received clinical acupuncture treatments for the relief of chronic low back or knee pain we found that those who had done well in treatment, i.e., good acupuncture responders, felt less pain with the experimental cold pressor pain stimulus than did those who had a poor clinical result. That is, those who had less clinical pain reduction felt the experimental pain more keenly. In this study hypnotic susceptibility and response to acupuncture were independent variables.

Acknowledgements. Collaborators in my research endeavors were: John Stern, Marjorie Brown, Sadashiv Parwatikar, Bernard Saletu, Monika Saletu, Ivan Sletten, Turan Itil, Ellen Itil, Sevket Akpinar, and Pacita Dy. This research was funded by a grant from the National Institutes of Health to the Missouri Institute of Psychiatry, University of Missouri School of Medicine, St. Louis, MO, Sept. 1972.

References

1. Mann F (1971) Atlas of Acupuncture. Heinemann, London
2. Brown ML, Ulett GA, Stern JA (1974) Acupuncture loci: techniques for location. Am J Chinese Med 2: 67-74
3. Shackel B (1959) Skin drilling. A method of diminishing galvanic skin potentials. Am J Psychol 72: 114
4. Liu YK, Varela M, Oswald R (1975) The correspondence between some motor points and acupuncture. Am J Chin Med 3: 347-358
5. Gunn CC Pain, acupuncture and related subjects. From: Worker's Compensation Board of British Columbia. Privately Published, 828 West Broadway, Vancouver, BC, V52IJ8
6. Brown ML, Ulett GA, Stern JA (1974) The effects of acupuncture on white blood cell counts. Am J Chin Med 2: 383-398
7. Cheng Tsung O (1973) Medicine in modern China. J Am Geriatr Soc 21 (7): 289-313
8. Chan P (1973) Wonders of Chinese Acupuncture. Borden, Alhambra USA
9. General Hospital of the Kwangchow Division PLA (1973) An inquiry into the analgesic principles of acupuncture anesthesia. (Abridged by John Kao.) Am J Chin Med 1: 172-176
10. Cracium T, Toma C (1973) Central nervous reactions after acupuncture. Am J Acupunct 1: 61-66
11. Cracium T, Toma C, Turdeanu V (1973) Neurohumoral modifications after acupuncture. Am J Acupunct 1: 67-70
12. Ulett AG, Perry SG (1974) Cytotoxic testing and leukocyte increase as an index to food sensitivity. Ann Allergy 33 (1): 23-32
13. Ward H, Reinhard E (1971) Chronic idiopathic leukocytosis. Ann Intern Med 75: 193-198
14. Spiegel H, Spiegel D (1978) Trance and Treatment. Basic Books, New York pp 370
15. Kroger WS (1972) Hypnotism and acupuncture. JAMA 220: 1012
16. Ulett GA, Peterson D (1965) Applied hypnosis and positive suggestion. Mosby, St. Louis
17. Orne MI, O'Connell DN (1967) Diagnostic ratings of hynotizability. Int J Exp Hypnosis 15: 125-133
18. Barber TX, Calverley PS (1963) Toward a theory of hypnotic behaviour: effects on suggestibility of task motivating instructions and attitudes towards hypnosis. J Abnorm Psychol 67: 557
19. Ulett GA, Akpinar S, Itil TM (1972) Hypnosis by videotape. Int J Clin Hypnosis 20: 46-91
20. Saletu B, Saletu M, Brown ML, Sletten IW, Ulett GA (1975) Hypno- and acupuncture analgesia: a neurophysiological reality? Neuropsychobiology 1: 281-242
21. Burch NR, Nettleton WJ, Sweeney J, Edwards RJ (1964) Period analysis of the electroencephalogram on a general purpose digital computer. Ann NY Acad Sci 155: 837-843
22. Shapiro D, Hsu W, Itil TM (1971) Period analysis of the EEG on the PDP-12. In: Wulfsohn, Scances (eds) The nervous system and electrical currents. Plenum, New York
23. Peking Acupuncture Anesthesia Coordinating Group (1973) Preliminary study on the mechanism of acupuncture anesthesia. Sci Sin [B] 16: 444-456
24. Chang, Hsiang-Tung (1974) Integrative action of the thalamus in the process of acupuncture for analgesia. Am J Chin Med 1: 61-72
25. Wall P (1972) An eye on the needle. New Scientist 55: 129-131
26. Wall P (1974) Acupuncture revisited. New Scientist 60: 31-34
27. Katz RL, Kao CX, Speigel H, Katz GT (1974) Acupuncture hypnosis. Adv Neurol 4: 819-825
28. Katz R (1973) (in Jenrick HP). Proceedings of the National Institutes of Health, Acupuncture Research Conference, Bethesda, MD, p 109
29. Lu Gwei-Djen, Needham J (1980) Celstial lancets. Cambridge University Press, pp 427

30. Omura Y (1975-1976) Editorial. Historical ascepts of acupuncture. Acupunct Electrother Res 1: 1-4, 17
31. Matsumoto T (1974) Acupuncture for physicians. Thomas, Springfield, p 204
32. Ulett GA (1983) Acupuncture is not hypnosis. Recent physiological studies. Am J Acupunct 11: 5-13
33. Goldstein A, Hilgard ER (1975) Failure of the opiate antagonist Naloxone to modify hypnotic analgesia. Proc Natl Acad Sci USA 72: 2031
34. Levine JD, Gordon NC, Fields HL (1978) The mechanism of placebo analgesia. Lancet 1: 654-657
35. Ulett GA (1982) Principles and practice of physiologic acupuncture. Green, St. Louis, pp 220
36. Ulett GA (1981) Acupuncture treatments for pain relief. JAMA 245: 768-769
37. Ulett GA (1984) Editorial. Acupuncture update - 1984. South Med J 78: 237-238
38. Ulett GA, Akpinar S, Itil TM (1972) Hypnosis - physiological, pharmacological reality. Am J Psychiatr 128 (7): 799-805

Appendix

Bruce Pomeranz

Acupuncture Analgesia for Chronic Pain:
Brief Survey of Clinical Trials

The papers reviewed below indicate that AA is very effective in treating chronic pain, helping 55%–85% of patients (compared to morphine which helps 70%). Secondly, these papers show that AA is better than placebo which helps only 30% of patients. These statements are based on evidence collected in four classes of studies (see recent reviews [15, 22, 25]).

Class A: studies in which there was no control group for comparison with the acupuncture group or in which there was a control group where the subjects received no treatment.

Class B: studies in which the control group received percutaneous acupuncture but at the wrong location (called sham acupuncture).

Class C: studies using a placebo control group (usually a disconnected TENS device or acupuncture needle taped to the skin). It is important to note that needles were not inserted percutaneously in the control group for class C studies and hence this is not considered to be sham acupuncture.

Class D: studies in which the control group received conventional therapy (e.g. drugs or physiotherapy).

In classes B and C, the experiments were single blind (the patients did not know about the sham or placebo, but the therapists knew). The quality of studies in descending order is class C, class D, class B and class A. Initially, it was thought that class B studies were similar in quality to those of class C. It was hoped that sham acupuncture (insertion of needles at wrong locations) was a good control for placebo effects and, hence, many studies were based on this approach. Unfortunately, experience has since shown that sham acupuncture helps 33%–50% of patients while placebo in class C helps only 30% of patients (note that true acupuncture helps 55%–85% of patients) [22, 25].

In the review by Lewith and Machin [15], it was convincingly argued that the statistical problems inherent in class B experiments, in which one group shows a 40% success rate (sham) and another group shows a 70% success rate (true acupuncture), make the burden of proof unrealistic, requiring at least 122 patients in the study to find a difference between the two groups. In contrast, placebos in class C only benefit 30% of patients, making the burden of proof easier. To compare 30% success in placebo controls with 70% success from true acupuncture requires only 70 patients. Hence, it is not surprising that two out of two studies [18, 20] in class C showed significant differences between treated and controls, whereas four out of six class B experiments failed to show differences [6, 7, 8, 26 no differences shown, 10, 19 differences shown]. Class B experiments should be repeated with larger sample size, above 122, to settle this problem.

Normally, we should completely ignore class A experiments as they are poorly controlled. This is too severe as most of these studies showed the 55%–85% success rate that we now know from class C experiments to be far above the placebo level of 30% [2, 3, 4, 5, 11, 12, 13, 14, 21, 23, 27].

Class D studies suffered from the same problems as class B, placing too big a burden of proof on the small sample size. Nevertheless, four of these studies did show AA to outperform the conventional medical treatment [9, 16, 17, 24] while one showed no difference [1] (perhaps due to a type II error).

However, even if the analgesic effects of acupuncture and of a chemical analgesic are equivalent, this is also a victory for AA, given the many side effects of analgesic drugs and the relatively few side effects of acupuncture.

Hence, from the above considerations, it is clear that AA helps from 55%–85% of patients which compares favorably with morphine (but with fever side effects). It works better than placebo; but more research is needed to see if it works better than sham acupuncture.

References

1. Ahonen E, Hakumaki M et al (1983) Acupuncture and physiotherapy in the treatment of myogenic headache patients: Pain relief and EMG activity. In: Bonica JJ (ed) Advances in pain research and therapy, vol 5. Raven Press, New York, pp 571–576
2. Chen GS (1977) Therapeutic effect of acupuncture for chronic pain. Am J Chin Med 5: 45–61
3. Cheng ACK (1975) The treatment of hedaches employing acupuncture. Am J Chin Med 3: 181–185
4. Coan RM, Wong G et al (1980) The acupuncture treatment of low back pain: a randomized controlled study. Am J Chin Med 8: 181–189
5. Coan RM, Wong G, Coan PL (1982) The acupuncture treatment of neck pain: a randomized controlled study. Am J Chin Med 9: 326–332
6. Edelist G, Gross AE, Langer F (1976) Treatment of low back pain with acupuncture. Can Anaesth Soc J 23: 303–306
7. Gaw AC, Chang LW, Shaw LC (1975) Efficacy of acupuncture on osteoarthritis pain. N Engl J Med 21: 375–378
8. Ghia J, Mao W, Toomey T, Gregg J (1976) Acupuncture and chronic pain mechanisms. Pain 2: 285–299
9. Gunn CC, Milbrandt WE et al (1980) Dry needling to muscle motor points for chronic low back pain. Spine 5: 279–291
10. Hansen PE, Hansen JH (1983) Acupuncture treatment of chronic facial pain: a controlled cross-over trial. Headache 23: 66–69
11. Kim KC, Yount RA (1974) The effect of acupuncture on migraine headache. Am J Chin Med 2: 407–411

12. Laitinen J (1975) Acupuncture for migraine prophylaxis: a prospective clinical study with six months follow-up. Am J Chin Med 3: 271–274
13. Lee PK, Andersen TW et al (1975) Treatment of chronic pain with acupuncture. J Am Med Assoc 232: 1133–1135
14. Leung PC (1979) Treatment of low back pain with acupuncture. Am J Chin Med 7: 372–378
15. Lewith GT, Machin D (1983) On the evaluation of the clinical effects of acupuncture. Pain 16: 111–127
16. Loh L, Nathan PW et al (1984) Acupuncture versus medical treatment for migraine and muscle tension headaches. J Neurol Neurosurg Psychiatry 47: 333–337
17. Loy TT (1983) Treatment of cervical spondylosis. Med J Aust 2: 32–34
18. MacDonald AJR, Macrae KD et al (1983) Superficial acupuncture in the relief of chronic low back pain. Ann R Coll Surg Engl 65: 44–46
19. Matsumoto T, Levy B, Ambruso V (1974) Clinical evaluation of acupuncture. Am Surg 40: 400–405
20. Petrie JP, Langley GB (1983) Acupuncture in the treatment of chronic cervical pain. A pilot study. Clin Exp Rheumatol 1: 33–35
21. Pontinen PJ (1979) Acupuncture in the treatment of low back pain and sciatica. Acupunct Electrother Res Int J 4: 53–57
22. Richardson PH, Vincent CA (1986) Acupuncture for the treatment of pain: a review of evaluative research. Pain 24: 15–40
23. Spoerel W (1976) Acupuncture in chronic pain. Am J Chin Med 4: 267–279
24. Sung YF, Kutner MH et al (1977) Comparison of the effects of acupuncture and codeine on postoperative dental pain. Anesth Analg 56: 473–478
25. Vincent CA, Richardson PH (1986) The evaluation of therapeutic acupuncture: concepts and methods. Pain 24: 1–13
26. Yue SJ (1978) Acupuncture for chronic back and neck pain. Acupunct Electrother Res Int J 3: 323–324
27. Yuen RWM, Vaughan RJ et al (1976) The response to acupuncture therapy in patients with chronic disabling pain. Med J Aust 1: 862–865

The Standard
Textbook

G. Stux, Düsseldorf; **B. Pomeranz,** Toronto

Acupuncture

Textbook and Atlas

1987. 98 figures and an acupuncture selector.
XI, 342 pages. Hard cover. ISBN 3-540-17331-5

Since its publication this book has become the standard text in acupuncture. The scientific basis of acupuncture is presented by Bruce Pomeranz, an eminent neurophysiologist who is in the vanguard of basic research in acupuncture. Following an introduction to the philosophical and theoretical background of traditional Chinese medicine, the traditional diagnostic system is presented in a manner easily comprehensible for the Western physician. The system of organs and channels with the 160 most important acupuncture points is depicted with localisation, indications and type of needling. The various techniques of needling, needle stimulation, needle material as well as moxibustion are covered at length. Following the presentation of the most important rules and principles for point selection there is a detailed description of the treatment of disorders with the essential acupuncture points and information on their stimulation.
Furthermore, there are clear chapters on ear, scalp and hand acupuncture, acupressure, and laser therapy.
A comprehensive glossary with translations of Chinese ideograms and point names completes the book.

Contents:
- Scientific Basis of Acupuncture
- Background and Theory of Traditional Chinese Medicine
- Diagnosis in Traditional Chinese Medicine
- Chinese System of Channels, Organs and Points
- Systematic Description of Channels and Points
- Regions with Important Acupuncture Points
- Technique of Acupuncture
- Moxibustion – Laser Acupuncture
- Ear Acupuncture – Acupressure
- Scalp and Hand Acupuncture
- Acupuncture Treatment of Different Diseases.

Springer-Verlag Berlin
Heidelberg New York London
Paris Tokyo Hong Kong

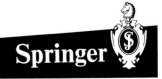

Springer

The compact introduction

G. Stux, B. Pomeranz

Basics of Acupuncture

1988. 63 figures. XI, 272 pages.
Soft cover. ISBN 3-540-19336-7

Basics of Acupuncture provides an introduction and quick reference for students and practitioners. It begins with a review of the scientific basis of acupuncture and relevant research. An introduction to the philosophy and theory of traditional Chinese medicine is then followed by a detailed account of diagnosis and description of the Chinese system of channels, functional organs, and points. The remainder of the book is devoted to treatment, based on Western modes of diagnosis. The methods and applications of needling and moxibustion are described, and the most important acupuncture points are given for frequently encountered diseases. This section is designed to teach the reader the underlying rules for point selection.
Basics of Acupuncture is a unique introduction book: for the first time Western science and medicine are combined with traditional Chinese concepts.
This compact paperback book is an abbreviated version of the comprehensive book entitled **Acupuncture, Textbook and Atlas.**

German editions:

G. Stux, N. Stiller, R. Pothmann, A. Jayasuriya

Akupunktur

Lehrbuch und Atlas

2., überarbeitete Auflage. 1985, Nachdruck 1987.
Gebunden. ISBN 3-540-15836-7

G. Stux

Grundlagen der Akupunktur

2., ergänzte Auflage. 1988. Broschiert.
ISBN 3-540-19172-0

Springer-Verlag Berlin
Heidelberg New York London
Paris Tokyo Hong Kong

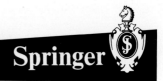